Type 2 Diabetes Pioneer

The No-Drug Success Story That
Keeps Getting Better Year after Year

TANYA ISCH CAYLOR

and BONAPARTE C. DAMOCLES

DEDICATION

This book is dedicated to Arnold C. Damocles,
his parents' Guardian Angel and an inspiration to all who met him.

CONTENTS

DISCLAIMER

Readers of this book should note that Bonny Damocles' no-drug solution for living well with type 2 diabetes may not work for everyone. Certainly it should not be attempted without first seeking medical advice from your doctor. It should be noted that Damocles began his experiment with his doctor's approval – and only after taking a cardiac stress test to determine whether his heart could endure strenuous exercise. Those who are already taking medication should not stop taking it without their doctor's consent.

HOW TO READ THIS BOOK

If you are the type of person who is disciplined enough to simply get the information you need and put it into action, then turn to Page 98, read "Bonny's Rules for Living Like You Have No Diabetes," and get to work implementing these guidelines into your new lifestyle.

If you act on his guidelines, then even reading those two pages will easily be worth the cost of this book – because you will save a MINIMUM of hundreds of dollars in your first year of learning to deal with type 2 diabetes. And the savings will increase exponentially from there with every passing year that you experience good health with zero complications or prescription drug costs.

If you would prefer to focus on a summary of how and why Bonny implemented his diabetes-management plan and how it evolved over time, turn to Section Two, "A New Challenge: Diabetes."

Finally, if you are the type of person who learns best while getting immersed in a story – "walking a mile in someone else's shoes" to gain insights and perspective gleaned from how he overcame the obstacles in his life – then start at the beginning and read through to the end.

In the process, you may learn a bit about chess, overcoming tragedy and heartache to find prosperity and happiness, the keys to a successful 59-year marriage, and why Bonny believes that the most selfless acts of kindness and compassion are rooted in selfish behavior.

However you choose to experience this book, thanks for reading – and good luck on your journey.

A PIONEER'S QUEST

In 1991, Bonny Damocles embarked on a quest to treat his type 2 diabetes without drugs, using exercise and healthy food as his only medicine.

Though his results were impressive enough to earn his doctor's approval, he was forging a path into an unknown future. He had no role models to follow. There were no Internet forums to compare notes with others.

He was on his own.

It was a role the Filipino immigrant was used to. Growing up in Manila, ashamed of his family's poverty, he was an outsider who stood on the sidelines, watching others for clues on how to improve the outcomes of seemingly hopeless situations.

Damocles did not fear diabetes. Compared with other challenges he had faced in his life – fleeing Japanese invasion forces during World War II, earning an engineering degree with almost no funding, stubbornly pursuing his dream of immigrating to America despite years of setbacks, and coming to terms with the terrible disease that eventually killed his youngest son – the prospect of tackling type 2 diabetes did not strike him as hopeless at all.

If anything, he was relieved to hear his diagnosis. He had feared his sudden, rapid weight loss might have been a sign of cancer.

At 55, after decades of using his wits to find a way around the most unsurmountable obstacles, Damocles was dubious of taking the most obvious path in life. In his experience, what looked like the easy way out of any situation almost always came boobytrapped with unpleasant surprises. From his perspective, looking at the prescriptions his doctor was writing out for him, he couldn't help wondering what new problems they would introduce even as they purportedly "fixed" his high blood sugar.

Damocles thought he knew what had caused his diabetes. It was the same thing that was happening to so many other Filipino immigrants he knew. After spending most of his life eating mostly plant foods and fish, walking everywhere he needed to go, in America he had abruptly switched to eating fast food and driving everywhere. Could he solve his problem by going back to the kind of diet and active lifestyle he'd been used to in the Philippines?

His doctor gave him two weeks to try his experiment. When he brought his blood sugar down more than 300 points in 10 days, his doctor gave him permission to continue doing things "his way."

Now, more than a quarter-century later, Damocles' simple regimen of diet, exercise and common sense continues to keep both his weight and his blood sugar in check. More importantly, it has helped him avoid the trademark complications of the disease.

At 81, he has more energy than he did before his diagnosis, jogging up the stairs in his home for 15 minutes four times each day. He frequently exercises barefoot, revealing feet that are shockingly nimble for a man who has had diabetes for nearly one-third of his life. He does not wear glasses, even when he drives.

Since Damocles' diagnosis, type 2 diabetes has exploded into a national epidemic. Type 2 diabetes now affects more than 29 million Americans. Every 23 seconds a new case is diagnosed – and many more go undiagnosed. One-fourth of all Americans over age 65 have this disease. It is the seventh leading cause of death in this country, and that's not even counting the cases in which it's considered a contributing factor.

Metformin, the drug most often used to treat type 2 diabetes, is now the most prescribed drug on the planet. Insulin, used to treat more advanced cases of type 2 diabetes, has skyrocketed in price, now costing patients hundreds of dollars per month. Though it helps control patients' blood sugar, it often leads to weight gain, thereby perpetuating the very problem it attempts to solve.

If Damocles had simply gone along with the usual way of doing things, passively accepting the prescriptions his doctor wrote out for him in 1991, it's hard to say what condition he would be in now. It's unlikely he could possibly be in better physical health than he is now – and he almost certainly would be worse off financially. According to the American Diabetes Association, people with diabetes incur average medical costs of $13,700 per year, with well over half that amount directly attributable to diabetes. The economic impact on the United States alone is estimated at $245 billion a year.

Today type 2 diabetes is widely viewed as a progressive disease that's only likely to get worse, both in individual cases and as a society. And yet Damocles has found it a relatively simple problem to fix. Given his experience, he often wonders why others are so reluctant to follow his lead.

He admits his journey has not always been easy. With no one to guide him, especially in those early years, he had to work through challenges using experimentation and ingenuity, the primary tools of pioneers in every field.

And yet, in many ways it has been much easier than most people imagine. By simply setting up and then maintaining a way of life based on a few good habits, Damocles has been able to enjoy life in ways that might not have been possible if he had never been diagnosed with diabetes in the first place.

Thanks to the Internet, gathering information on type 2 diabetes has never been easier. And yet even now, Damocles only rarely encounters others who have embarked on similar journeys. Those who do are often afraid to eat carbohydrates, even those that come from whole plant foods. Though studies are now beginning to validate what Damocles and others have proven through personal experience, many diabetes forums remain a hostile environment for those who choose to try diet and exercise as their only medication.

"I was met with a lot of negativity on the forums by people who believe the only path to control is meds," wrote Damocles' friend Anna, a nurse whom he met online after her diagnosis in 2007. "What we do is not magic, it's just common sense. It *does* work for us. While others might not have as much success, and might need meds to gain control, I do believe there are others like us out there."

This is Damocles' story of the ongoing journey he began in 1991 and the path he's been exploring ever since, generating results that continue to please his doctors while saving him money. He has yet to encounter anyone else on the planet who has gone more than a quarter century successfully controlling type 2 diabetes without drugs. And yet he's convinced that if more people tried his method, the success he's enjoyed would be commonplace.

Damocles' no-drug solution for living well with type 2 diabetes may not work for everyone. Certainly it should not be attempted without first seeking medical advice from your doctor. It should be noted that Damocles began his experiment with his doctor's approval, and only after taking a cardiac stress test to determine whether his heart could endure strenuous exercise. Those who are already taking medication should not stop taking it without their doctor's consent.

But it is never too late to help your body control blood sugar the way it was designed to, with diet and exercise. If you have recently received a diagnosis of type 2 diabetes, or have been told you have prediabetes, now is the time to act. Damocles' story can provide hope and motivation, no matter where you are in your own journey.

When it comes to type 2 diabetes, in a sense *everyone* is a pioneer. This is a disease that forces you to leave your old way of life behind. We may live in a land where rich foods are plentiful and most people can easily avoid hard physical labor, but there is no drug on earth that enables a person with diabetes to continue overeating and leading a sedentary lifestyle without suffering debilitating physical complications and shortening their life.

Regardless of whether you use insulin or diabetes medications, you *will* be forced to leave your usual routine behind – or suffer the consequences.

Your new way of life will force you to figure out which foods raise your blood sugar and what type of exercise you like well enough to stick with it. If you don't, you will pay the price in compromised health and an earlier death – regardless of whether you use diabetes medications or not.

But as Damocles and others have learned, the life of a diabetes pioneer need not be difficult, expensive or miserable. In fact, you may find – as he did – that your best years are yet to come.

I. LEARNING TO SURVIVE

A TOUGH CHILDHOOD

It may seem like a cruel joke that someone who endured starvation as a child, growing up in the Japanese-occupied Philippines during World War II, could end up with a disease associated with overeating and a sedentary lifestyle.

But it makes perfect sense to Bonaparte C. Damocles. The way he sees it, overindulging after having finally arrived in the "Land of Plenty" – achieving his lifelong dream of reaching the United States – was a natural reaction to the deprivation he experienced as a child.

Bonny, as he prefers to be called, was 5 years old when the Japanese invaded his country on Dec. 8, 1941, the day after the attack on Pearl Harbor. He and his family joined a procession of thousands as they fled Manila, walking several days to reach Cabanatuan City, about 61 miles away.

In his youth, long before Bonny was born, his father had taken a bicycling trip around the main island of the Philippines. Though Mariano C. Damocles was a young man from a prosperous family, he relied on the good-natured hospitality of his fellow Filipinos when he needed food or lodging. Now, decades later, the residents of Cabanatuan City were equally generous, sharing food with the camping refugees as U.S. and Filipino forces battled the Japanese farther south. But this time, the circumstances were very different. With two young children in tow, Bonny's parents had managed to salvage only a few possessions. No one knew when, or if, they could return to Manila.

On April 9, 1942, U.S. forces lost the Bataan Peninsula, giving the Japanese Imperial Army control of the main island of Luzon. As 75,000 captured American and Filipino soldiers embarked on what later became known as the Bataan Death March, in which thousands died or were killed, the Japanese ordered the civilian evacuees at Cabanatuan City and other refugee camps to return to their cities of origin. Bonny and his family rode a bus back to Manila.

Life was much different under Japanese rule. The college near his family's apartment, the University of Santo Tomas, had been converted into a prison camp. Because there was a news blackout during the duration of the war, he never knew what transpired there – or anywhere else, for that matter. He and his relatives never learned the fate of a cousin who disappeared while serving in the Philippine Army. All they knew was that times were tough – and food was scarce.

"Lack of food for us during the war happened on more than one occasion," Bonny recalls. "Nearly all Filipinos then were just skin and bones. The Japanese who occupied our country for four years got most of the food that was supposed to be for Filipinos."

As Bonny's family sometimes went days at a time with nothing to eat, he learned to fill his stomach with water.

"Did I faint? No. I was supposed to, I think, but the truth is, I never did. Why? Maybe because of the so-called survival instinct in me."

At one point, while his family was living with his mother's cousins – one of whose husbands had a

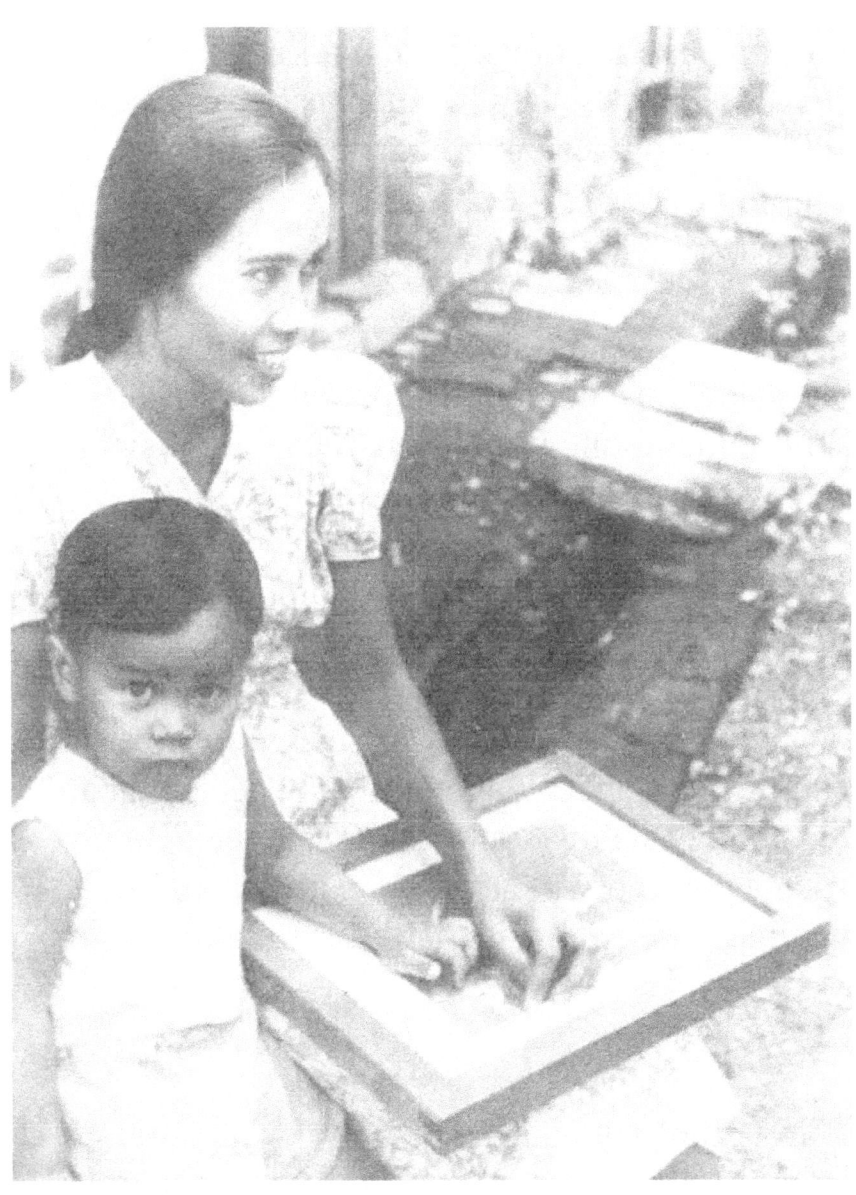

Bonny and his mother, Maria Corpuz Damocles, in the days before World War II came to the Philippines.

bit of meager earnings from working for the Japanese army – they lived on rice that had been salvaged from a sunken Japanese cargo ship. Filipino divers found tons of rice in the shipwreck. Though it had been submerged in seawater, bags were brought ashore, where it became known as 'sisid rice. (In Tagalog, the language most commonly spoken in the Philippines along with English, the term 'sisid literally translates as "underwater diving.")

"It was edible, but did not taste good," Bonny recalls.

Whatever food they had was shared equally, but carefully rationed and kept in a locked cupboard. One night, feeling "unbearable hunger," Bonny used a pin to pry the lock open and filled his shrunken stomach with handfuls of tainted rice.

***

During the years of the Japanese occupation, Bonny learned to stay close to home. In a large city like Manila, it's not like there were soldiers on every street corner. They were primarily clustered in strategic locations, such as government buildings, police precincts, Malacanang Palace and the prison camp at the

University of Saint Tomas. Still, he heard stories about the Japanese beheading Filipinos they suspected of being associated with the guerilla movement.

No evidence was necessary. Even worse, some Filipinos, desperate for food or money, were rumored to be informing on their countrymen for economic gain.

"We called them 'makapili' (traitors)," Bonny said. "What they did to hide their identities was to cover their heads with paper bags with two holes for them to see and point out to the Japs other Filipinos they wanted beheaded. No questions were asked by the enemies. They would just get their machete and kill."

Later, when he went to work for the Manila City Engineer's Office, Bonny met a supervisor who showed him marks on the back of his head.

"He said that he was a beheading survivor during the war."

***

One night in early February 1945, Bonny and his father were walking home from visiting his father's relatives. Suddenly they heard gunfire. It went on and on and on. In the dark, it was hard to know how close it was or exactly what was happening.

"We did not know what to do," Bonny said. "Luckily, a homeowner allowed us to take cover in his house."

They stayed in the stranger's home until the next day, when the shooting stopped. When they emerged from the house, "we saw many people in the streets celebrating the arrival of the Americans."

When he evacuated the Bataan Peninsula in a PT boat in 1942, General Douglas MacArthur had vowed "I shall return." The United States, which had made the Philippines a commonwealth in 1936 and promised independence a decade later, had continued supplying the Filipino resistance during the war. By October 1944 MacArthur and his American troops had come ashore on the island of Leyte. Now, though pockets of Japanese soldiers would continue battling until the end of the war that August, U.S. forces had pushed into Manila.

Bonny's family was thrilled. But their troubles were far from over.

***

Mariano C. Damocles was still a young man when he became heavily involved in the Methodist Church. Eventually he became one of about 50 Filipino deacons in a country that remained primarily Roman Catholic – including most of his own family. But he was not good with money. Even before the Japanese invasion, he had used up his inheritance.

For Bonny, all that remained of his family's privileged past was his name. In a country where Spanish surnames are the norm – a reflection of four centuries of colonial rule – Bonny's surname came from an ancient parable told by the Roman philosopher Cicero. In "The Sword of Damocles," a tyrannical and paranoid king grants a foolish flatterer the trappings of royalty. Distracted by his good fortune, Damocles at first does not notice that above his head a sword hangs by a very thin thread – a reflection of the king's perspective on the perils of power.

Whatever message Bonny's ancestors intended to send by taking the name Damocles, the fact that they were even aware of the tale was a sign of a privileged background. "Only the wealthy Filipinos could afford to get a higher education during the four centuries of Spanish rule," he said.

Having grown up in luxury, pursuing interests that had little to do with either the acquisition of or retention of wealth, Bonny's father "was already a very poor religious man" by the time he married Bonny's mother.

Maria Corpuz Damocles, Mariano's second wife, was 20 years younger than he was, and just as poor. They lived in a house divided into four apartments with Maria's relatives.

"We were the only one whose electricity was disconnected every now and then because my dad could not pay the monthly electric bill," Bonny recalls. "When we had no light, I had to go to a Chinese store to do my school homework."

While Mariano tended to the church and a small photography business that failed to pay the bills, Bonny's mother washed other families' clothes to help out.

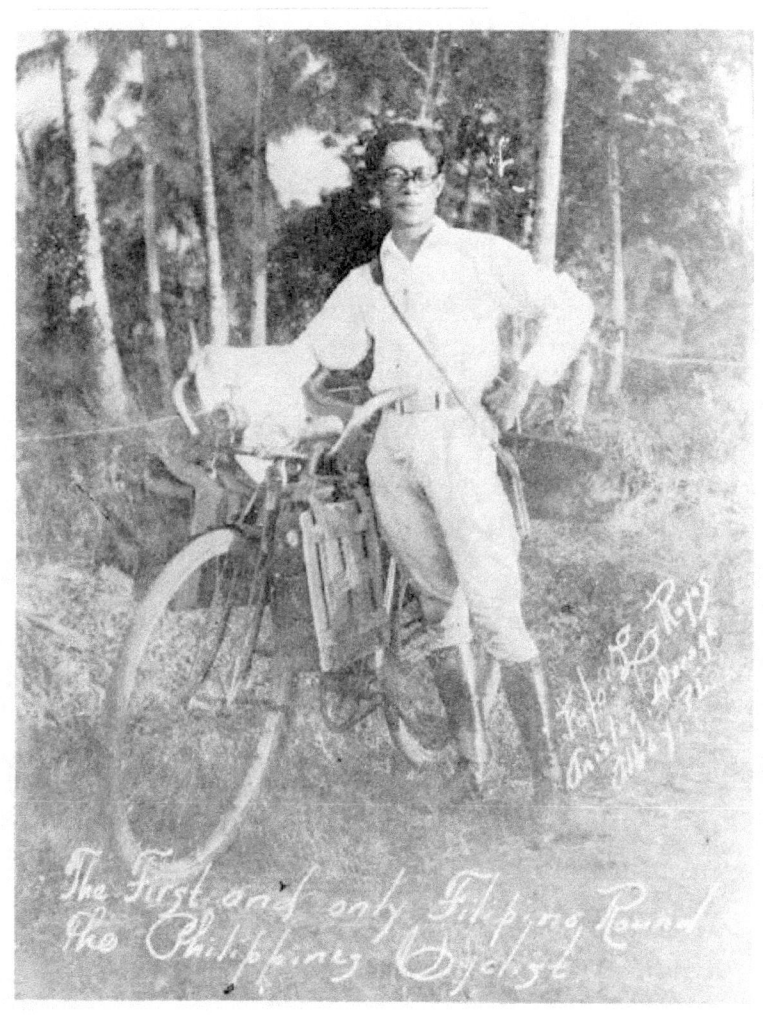

The First and only Filipino Round
the Philippines Cyclist

Bonny's father, Mariano C. Damocles, toured the big island of the Philippines by bicycle in his youth.

At Christmas, when Filipino children went door to door asking for Christmas gifts, Bonny quickly learned his best bet was to visit his wealthy Roman Catholic relatives. On Christmas Day, these same relatives provided food and gifts for all of the children who attended a large family gathering.

"Not once did our family contribute to the celebration expenses," Bonny recalls. "We were very poor."

At school, he learned to go off by himself as the other children ate their lunches. More often than not, he had nothing. "I did not like to feel miserable watching others munching something."

An uncle who worked at the Department of Education wanted to help his sister's family, so he sent Bonny's mother to school to study teaching. After Maria earned her diploma, her brother found her a teaching job in Surigao del Norte, a province in Mindanao. Because it was far from their home, Bonny only saw his mother when she returned during her two-month summer vacation.

During all four years of high school, "I had no mother," he says. With little to eat and only two shirts and two pairs of pants that he nonetheless made sure to keep clean, Bonny felt isolated from his classmates.

"I was a loner and getting to be very good at it," he recalls. "I learned how to observe people from a distance. I learned from their body language, their actions, their mannerisms. I became a sort of expert on people's behavior."

Then, during his sophomore year, a classmate taught him and another boy to play chess. It was a life-changing experience. Chess was a perfect game for a boy who was used to quietly studying others and making observations about their motivations, successes and failures. The chess board was a safe place to try out ideas and strategies of his own. It also gave him his first true friend, as he and the other beginning chess student, Magdiwang Recato – Diwang for short – embraced the game.

During their summer vacation in 1955, Diwang and Bonny and another classmate participated in the first Junior National Chess Championship tournament in Manila. None of them won a prize. But simply having the opportunity to participate – and in the process, securing a three-week job moving chess pieces on a display board so the audience could see which moves the competitors were making – gave Bonny newfound confidence.

Later in life, Bonny would credit chess with giving him a framework for working out problems and finding shortcuts that has helped him in countless ways.

"Chess has taught me to think, talk and act like I know more than I actually do, to accomplish more in less time, spend less for more important things, and stay healthier by eating less and exercising more," he says.

But even in high school, the lessons he learned on the chess board helped open his eyes to the fact that "there really are many possibilities in life, and having the luck to choose the right ones can make me truly happier than I should be."

Though Bonny was still too embarrassed by his poverty to risk getting to know any girls at his school, he and a few close friends often talked of their hopes and dreams. Having been educated in an American-style school system that emphasized the American language and way of life, perhaps it was not surprising that almost all of their plans revolved around someday finding their way to the United States.

"Nearly all of us wanted to try joining the U.S. Navy," Bonny recalls. Though two of his friends eventually became naval officers, he was never called for an interview.

After graduation, Diwang entered the Manuel L. Quezon University School of Engineering and Architecture. Bonny decided to pursue studies at an inexpensive government school, the Philippine College of Commerce. It was cheap, a short walk from his family's apartment, and provided training in classes such as typing, stenography, and economics that he thought would be helpful in finding a job.

At PCC, Bonny soon rose to the top of his class. Diwang, who sometimes dropped by for a game of chess, kept trying to talk his old friend into transferring to the engineering school, certain that Bonny's high grades could earn him a scholarship.

The following year, Bonny joined Diwang at MLQUSEA. It was a good move, he thought. Not only was he getting a superior education on scholarship, but he had more opportunities to play chess with his old friend. He also found a mentor: an English professor who had studied in the United States.

"He told us, his students, about how hard he worked in the U.S. to support himself. He worked in the stockroom. He being short, about 5 feet, and his American co-workers being taller and stronger, that meant that he had to work twice as hard as the others. He had to walk twice as fast to produce the same output as the others had."

Nonetheless, his professor's tales of life in the United States made living there sound like it was worth every inconvenience along the way. Bonny was not sure how or when he could make it happen, but he was more determined than ever to someday make it to America.

CHRISTMAS
ON ANOTHER PLANET

In retrospect, one of the best things that ever happened to Bonny was losing his scholarship at the Manuel L. Quezon University School of Engineering and Architecture.

At the time, just one semester into his schooling, it certainly didn't seem like a good development. He went to see his English professor, who was also the school registrar, to discuss his precarious situation. He knew he could not afford to continue his education without his scholarship.

"What skills do you have?" his professor asked. When Bonny replied that he could type and knew stenography, his professor agreed to hire him to work part-time in the registrar's office.

"You don't get any pay," the registrar said, "but you don't pay for your schooling."

Working in the registrar's office meant that Bonny spent a lot of time looking through students' records. He couldn't help noticing that a girl named Nemia Cambil was not only a consistent scholar at the university, but had previously been valedictorian of both her grade school and her high school. He asked Diwang to introduce him to this student. "You're looking at her right now," his friend replied, pointing out a young woman who was coming down the stairs toward them. But Diwang refused to introduce them, and Bonny was too shy to say anything.

Later, when Nemia began working part-time in the school library, Bonny saw his opportunity. Since they were now both school employees, he figured it was not unreasonable for him to try to get to know her. Six months later, on June 3, 1958, they got married.

It was a simple ceremony before a judge. Their families were poor, and Bonny's mother did not approve of them rushing into marriage at a time when they were not earning enough money to support themselves.

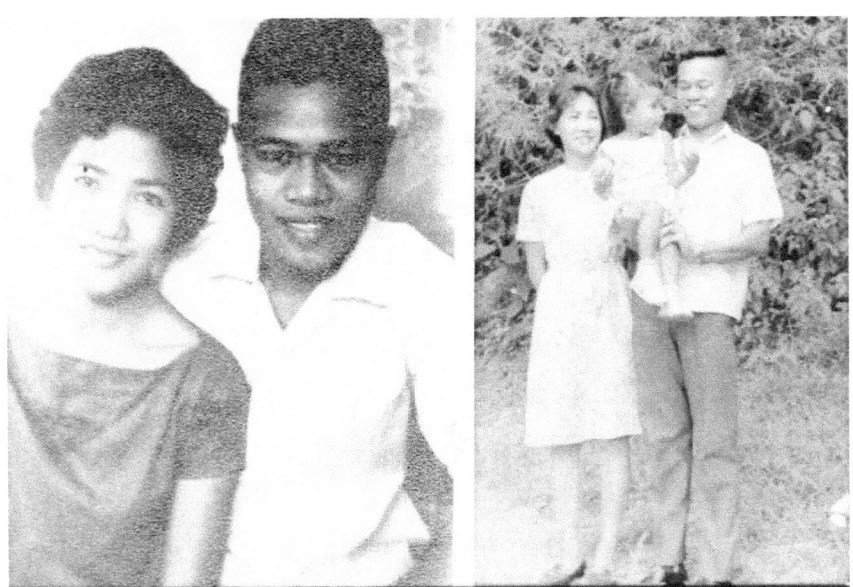

Bonny and Nemia the day after their wedding in 1958, left, and a few years later with their daughter, Arlene.

Bonny knew it seemed like a rash decision to his mother. But to a chess player, who was constantly studying the habits of others to figure out what made them successful, securing an intelligent life partner was a big priority. Having found what he wanted in Nemia, he explains, "I married her as fast as possible to eliminate the possibility of losing her to her other admirers."

The young couple lived with Bonny's parents while continuing their studies and working their part-time jobs. Their first child, Oral, was born in 1959.

"We are the only people, I think, who have never worn wedding rings," Bonny says. "We were too poor to afford them."

Eventually the young couple earned their engineering degrees, found better-paying jobs and moved into their own apartment. Over time they built a respectable life. Bonny became a management analyst in the Manila mayor's office, a job he was able to obtain with Diwang's help after his friend became the protege of a professor who was also the city engineer. Nemia, who started out teaching physics and working in government laboratories, eventually became supervising patent agent in the Philippines Patent Office. They had a maid and a nanny to help look after their four children.

But in the Philippines, a respectable job did not necessarily translate into a good income. And having household help was hardly a status symbol. Filipino maids worked for almost nothing. Bonny and Nemia could not afford to buy their children bicycles; securing a loan for a house or even a car was impossible. Bonny felt stuck, knowing neither of them were likely to

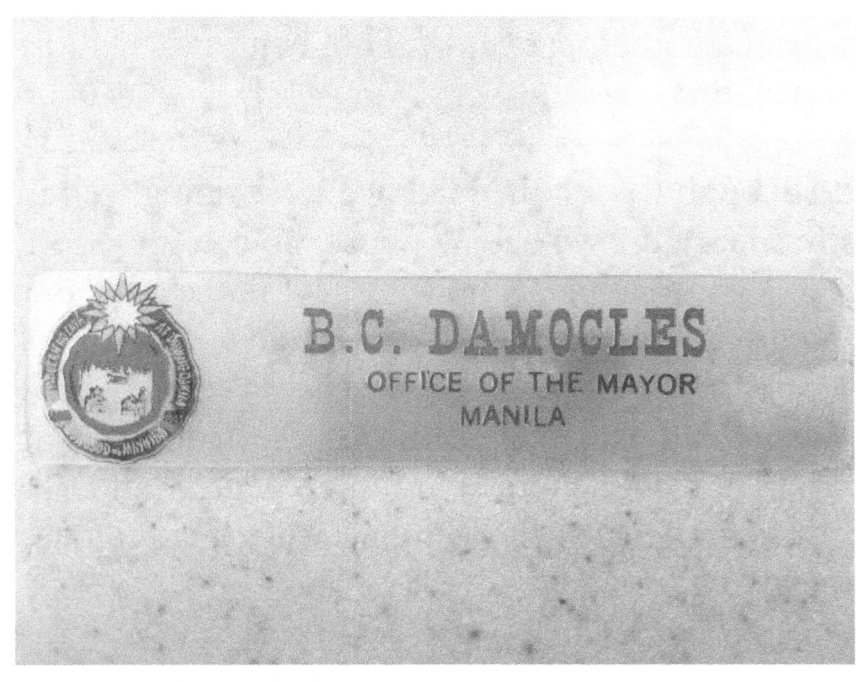

Bonny wore this name badge while working in the Manila Mayor's Office from 1965 to 1972. He credits Mayor Antonio J. Villegas with coming up with a better idea to replace the Philippine custom of celebrating the New Year with firecrackers, which often caused injuries and sometimes even death. "His idea was to put coins in a can and shake this can as fast and as vigorously as possible during the one-minute period when the old year changes into the new year, and at the same time pray for a better, healthier, and wealthier new year," Bonny recalls. "Since I heard this idea, we have been doing it every year." Like Bonny, Villegas eventually immigrated to America, where he later died in Reno, N.V.

advance in their careers without better connections.

"Although we felt then that we were doing well in life," he said, "we had no house, no car, no jewelry, no savings – none of anything except the big dream to reach the U.S. someday."

When that opportunity came, through a U.S. program that encouraged Filipino degree holders in certain fields such as engineering to immigrate, they went for it.

As a registered chemical engineer with extensive experience in reviewing patent applications, Nemia's application was approved first, in late 1968. But it wasn't until the summer of 1972 that U.S. Immigration and Naturalization Services allowed her to fly to Chicago to join a former co-worker from the patent office.

Bonny and their four children – Oral, Arlene, Carlo, and Arnold – arrived in October.

"Totally broke" – owing Northwest Airlines thousands of dollars for plane tickets in a "Fly Now, Pay Later" program – the five new arrivals crammed into the two-bedroom apartment where Nemia had been sharing space with her friend's family of six. But they were hardly discouraged. Nemia had helped arrange a job for Bonny at the same factory where she and their hosts were working. Soon they were earning far more money than they had ever made in their government jobs back home.

Suddenly every day was like Christmas – on another planet.

"Our first Christmas celebration in the U.S. started very early," Bonny recalls. "We left the Philippines on Oct. 18, 1972. We landed in Chicago O'Hare International Airport on the same day. The following day, there was snow everywhere. Our host told us to taste it. We did. That was the start of our new life, and also the beginning of our first Christmas celebration in the U.S."

Back in Manila, Christmas merrymaking began on Nov. 2 and lasted until Jan. 6. In their adopted country, with so much to celebrate and so many wonderful things so readily available, Bonny's family saw no reason to wait.

"We started buying American food we never had in the Philippines, like cheese, butter, bread, ham, sausage, grapes, apples, chocolate bars, and many other things," Bonny recalls. "We had no Christmas tree, but we had all kinds of gifts for ourselves like new clothes, new winter coats, boots, blankets, comforters, pillows. Everything we bought for ourselves was new. We learned to love fast food places, which did not exist in the Philippines."

One bright sunny day, heading out to shop for toys for the children, they were startled to discover that sunshine does not always bring warmth. The temperature that day was right around zero. "After less than a minute outdoors, we had to get back indoors as fast as we could!"

Everything happened quickly in their adopted country, it seemed. Before long, the owners of the apartment, Filipino relatives of Nem's former co-worker, moved to a new place and Bonny's family moved into the second-floor apartment they had occupied. Three months after Bonny and the children's arrival, the family bought their first car: a 1972 orange Volkswagen Super Beetle.

By the fall of 1973, after more than a year as a clerk to a shop foreman at Vapor Corp., Nemia found a position as a patent agent with the Union Carbide company. Bonny, who was working as an expediter for Vapor Corp.'s general foreman,

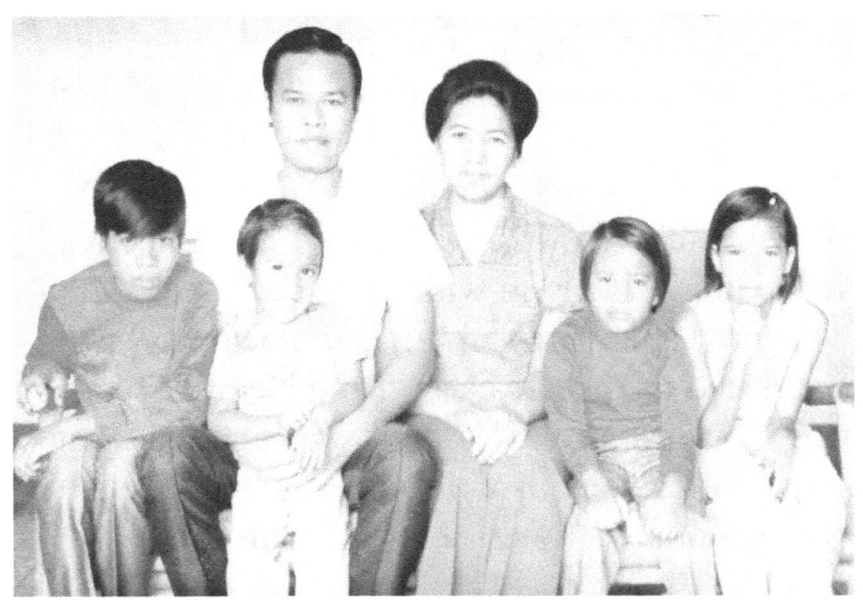

This photo of the Damocles family was taken about a month after they arrived in Chicago in 1972. From left: Oral, Arnold, Bonny, Nemia, Carlo, and Arlene.

stayed with the company because he found his boss to be kind and generous: "He never got tired of teaching me everything I should learn about manufacturing shop operations."

Bonny's loyalty was repaid when his boss was promoted.

"As a shop worker reporting directly to the vice president of operations, I could easily find the opportunity to talk with anybody in the company," he said. Soon he began playing chess with a top executive during his daily lunch break.

By 1976, the family bought a new home in the Chicago suburb of Bolingbrook, Ill. Eighteen years after moving in with Bonny's parents, they were now able to return the favor. Though his father had died years earlier, and Nemia's mother was now dead as well, Bonny was pleased – and surprised – when his wife suggested they help his mother come to America to live with them.

"My mom did not wholeheartedly welcome Nem when I brought her home," Bonny recalled. "Filipinos I grew up with in the Manila Metropolitan area were known for paying back in kind. There was no forgiving." It was yet another reminder, he says, that his wife was "one of a kind."

Bonny's mother arrived in late March of that year, about a week before a big snowstorm. "Upon seeing the big pile of snow in the street, she said that it was like the perennial floods in Manila. The only difference was that snow was white and the Manila floodwater was black." Though the former teacher would wind up working in a nursing home, she could not have been more thrilled.

"My mother, was very, very happy and very, very excited to reach the good old U.S.A.," Bonny said. "It is every Filipino's dream to see this great country."

Life was good. In the Land of Plenty, there were so many wonderful labor-saving devices – machines to wash and dry their clothes, cook their food and even clean their dishes – they did not even miss having a maid.

A BLESSING
IN A TERRIBLE DISGUISE

Bonny's family had been living in their new home in the suburbs less than one year when they received the shock of their lives: Their youngest son, Arnold, was not just going through a clumsy phase. Doctors told them he had Duchenne Muscular Dystrophy – a disease that progressively weakens the muscles, typically leading to death before age 20.

To say that Arnold's condition helped put Bonny's later diagnosis of type 2 diabetes in perspective is a gross understatement. There is simply no comparison between a fatal disease that strikes innocent children and a disease whose devastating effects can be warded off with simple lifestyle changes. But Bonny did learn courage and resolve from his youngest child, who surprised doctors by living to see not only his 20th birthday but his 30th as well.

In two framed photos of Arnold that now bear places of honor on Bonny and Nemia's fireplace mantel, one is a grinning boy around 9 years old and the other is a handsome 17-year-old who has just graduated from high school. In both head-and-shoulder portraits, there is no outward sign of what was happening to the youth's muscles. There is no flicker of sadness or disappointment on his face. And yet in the years between the time the photos were taken, Arnold suffered a heart attack and gradually lost the ability to walk. Eventually he would be unable to breathe on his own without a respirator. But he stayed positive throughout his life, which ended in 1999, about a month after his 31st birthday.

"You will not believe it if I tell you that my wife, our daughter and I – who worked very, very hard to make our son enjoy a happy, comfortable and long life – were not as sad as we were expected to be in losing him," Bonny says.

"The reason? During all the time that he was with us, we showed him the best love a human being can ever feel. Everything he asked for, even if we could not afford it, he miraculously got it.

"There was a time not long after he was diagnosed that he wanted an in-ground swimming pool. We told him that we could not afford it. Not long after that, my wife got an unexpected large bonus from her employer. So he and everybody else in the family were pleasantly surprised that an expensive swimming pool would become a part of our newly bought house in Bolingbrook, Illinois."

Arnold was already using a wheelchair when he had a heart attack, at age 15, in December 1983. No one, including Arnold, understood what was happening when he began to complain that his chest hurt. But the Muscular Dystrophy Medical Research Team at Hinsdale Hospital, which had been monitoring his case for six years, explained that his weakening heart muscle was to blame.

Arnold spent the holidays in the hospital that year. He never returned to school, earning his high school diploma with the help of a tutor who came to the family's home.

Nonetheless, the wheelchair-using teenager expressed the desire to travel. And once again, Arnold's wish came true.

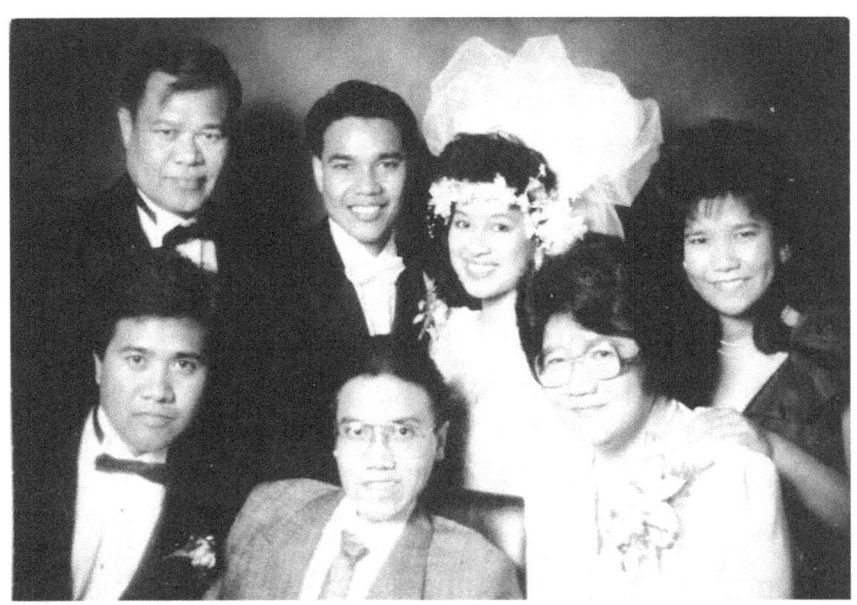

Arnold, front center, at his brother Carlo's wedding in July 1990, two days before his 22nd birthday. At the time, Arnold had already exceeded the average life expectancy of someone with Duchenne muscular dystrophy. He would eventually reach his 31st birthday. From upper left: Bonny, Carlo and his new wife Teresa, Arnold's sister Arlene. Front row: Arnold's brother Oral, Arnold and his mother, Nemia.

In 1986, the same year Arnold received his high school diploma, Nemia lost her job with Union Carbide. Within a few months, however, she found a job as a patent agent with the Dow Chemical Company in Midland, Mich. Bonny, Nemia, and Arnold decided to make the move. Bonny's mother, who had been helping to care for

Arnold, would stay behind in Bolingbrook, with Arnold's grown siblings and Bonny's brothers, Myriel and Pasteur and their families, who had also immigrated to the Chicago area.

Bonny, who had started an export business on the side, with the help of a cousin back in the Philippines and a helpful manager from Vapor Corp's international division, would work from home while taking care of Arnold.

In October 1987, Nemia's new employer asked her to attend a seminar in Germany. Bonny and Arnold decided to go along, with help from his brother Carlo and his girlfriend.

While they were sightseeing in Baden Baden, with Carlo pushing his brother's wheelchair, an American tourist asked Bonny how he could enjoy his vacation "with them tagging along."

"I was about to say, 'How could I enjoy my vacation if they were not with me?'" Bonny recalls. But he remained silent, wishing as usual to avoid confrontation.

Arnold treasured his trip of a lifetime. But in his remaining years, as his body became increasingly difficult to handle, he shifted his focus to what he could do to impact the lives of others. The most obvious focal point was the Jerry Lewis telethon to raise money for the Muscular Dystrophy Association. The MDA had proved extremely helpful to Arnold over the years, and every year Arnold asked his parents to make a donation in hopes of helping others, as well as funding research that might someday lead to a cure.

But Arnold's interest in helping others didn't stop there. Whenever he saw something on television or his computer that caught his interest, a way that he thought his family could help someone, he begged his parents to do what they could. Bonny and Nemia began to call it "Arnold's Game." And through Arnold's interest in studying the stock market, he was able to generate some income to help fund his projects.

One of Arnold's final projects before his death on Aug. 29, 1999, was to help inspire a program to bring eight jobless Filipinos to America to perform seasonal work at a hotel on Mackinac Island. Earlier that year, when one of Bonny's college classmates was visiting them in Midland, Bonny saw a newspaper article on a hotel that used Jamaican labor during the tourist season.

In discussing the article with his classmate, who was in the construction business, both men wondered about the possibility of bringing over Filipinos to do the same kind of work. Arnold, who by this time had been on a respirator for several years, nodded and smiled at the idea.

As far as Bonny was concerned, the decision was made.

"Who is the father who would not do his best to make his sick son happy forever?" he asks.

"The first wave of jobless Filipinos got to meet Arnold on their way to Mackinac Island. On their way back home, Arnold was already gone."

But Arnold's Game continued even after Arnold left them. Over the next two years, more than 100 unemployed Filipinos – many of them descendants of Bonny's aunts, who never received their share of the inheritance his father squandered – got an opportunity to do seasonal work at hotels in both Mackinac Island and in Colorado Springs, Colo.

"I bet Arnold smiles every time I tell that story," Bonny says. "Nem and I like to say that Arnold's Game will continue for as long as we live."

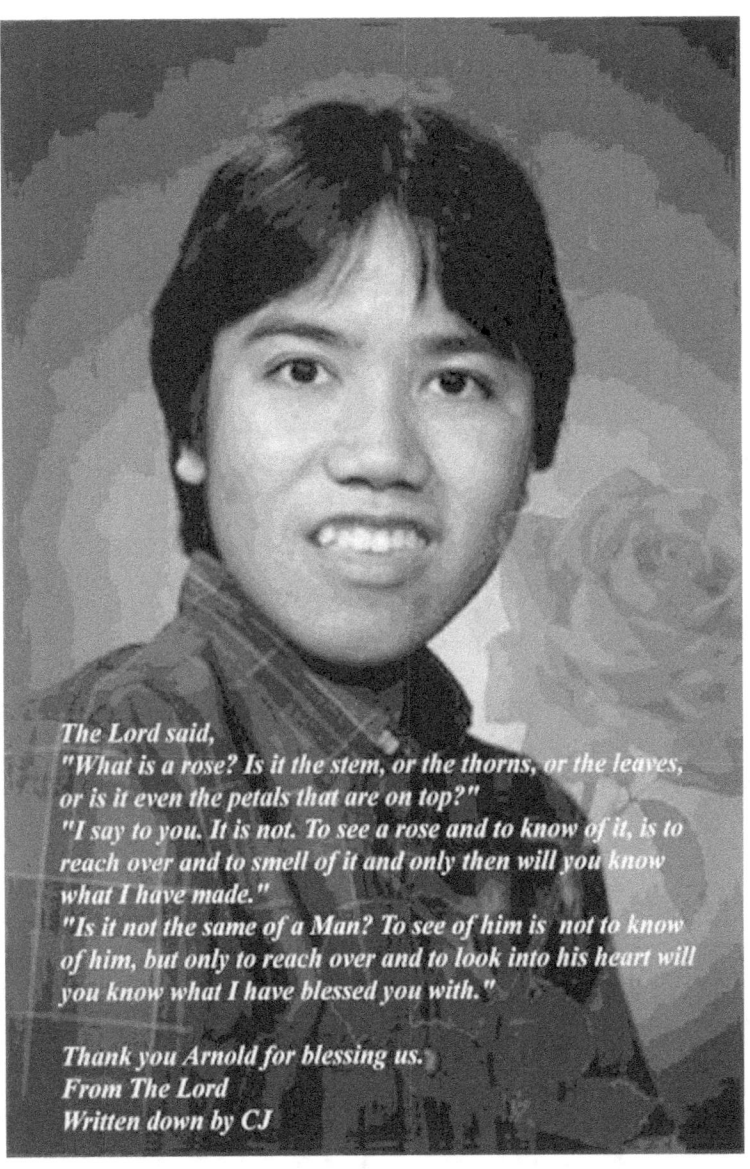

The Lord said,
"What is a rose? Is it the stem, or the thorns, or the leaves, or is it even the petals that are on top?"
"I say to you. It is not. To see a rose and to know of it, is to reach over and to smell of it and only then will you know what I have made."
"Is it not the same of a Man? To see of him is not to know of him, but only to reach over and to look into his heart will you know what I have blessed you with."

Thank you Arnold for blessing us.
From The Lord
Written down by CJ

Arnold Damocles died in 1999, about a month and a half after his 31st birthday.

II. A NEW CHALLENGE: DIABETES

LEARNING TO LIVE IN REVERSE

When Bonny and his family immigrated to the United States in 1972, the 37-year-old carried less than 130 pounds on his 5 foot, 7 inch frame.

Not surprisingly, given the dramatic changes in his diet, he began to put on weight.

"Where we came from, we seldom ate chicken, beef and pork because they were expensive," he said. "We had no pizza and no packaged foods like corn chips and tortillas. We ate mostly leafy vegetables, dried beans, fish, nuts, fruits, seaweed, canned sardines, canned salmon, and once in a long while, canned corned beef."

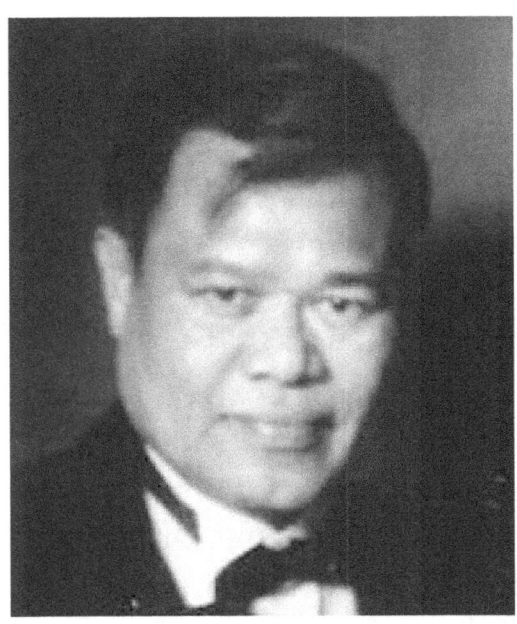

After living in America for nearly 20 years, Bonny had put on more than 35 pounds.

In America, with both parents working and no household staff to do the cooking, as they had been used to back home, Bonny and Nemia relied on cheap and plentiful fast food to keep their family fed. When they placed a takeout order at Kentucky Fried Chicken or Burger King, they ordered enough food to last for multiple meals, plus snacks.

Bonny wasn't overly concerned when his weight crept up over the years to 165 pounds. This was what it must feel like, he thought, to be a well-fed American.

But when he suddenly lost 20 pounds within two weeks in 1991, despite nearly constant hunger, he feared he had cancer. By then his family had been courageously coping with the knowledge of Arnold's deadly disease for several years. What would happen if Bonny, as Arnold's primary caregiver, got sick or even died?

Bonny's doctor questioned him on what other symptoms he was experiencing. Upon hearing of his excessive thirst, frequent urination, blurred vision and leg cramps, his doctor told him he doubted cancer was the problem.

Under the circumstances, "I was very, very happy to learn I had type 2 diabetes instead," Bonny recalls.

It wasn't hard to see how it had happened: He had gone from being a person who once walked everywhere he went to someone with almost no physical activity at all. He had always been a heavy eater. But instead of filling up on fruit, vegetables, rice and seafood, for years now he'd been gorging himself on pizza, hot dogs, fried chicken, potato chips, and a favorite from his early days in Chicago, big beef sandwiches with jalapeno peppers.

The question was, what was he going to do about it?

After his doctor got his lab tests back, he called to tell Bonny to report to his office right away so he could get started on prescription medications to help control his blood sugar. But Bonny, who had been quizzing a neighbor with diabetes, had learned that this man's medication had given him problems with hypoglycemia, or low blood sugar. In his neighbor's opinion, this was almost worse than the high blood sugar the medication was supposed to correct.

"I decided that was not for me," Bonny said. "I determined to avoid all medications if possible."

In Bonny's mind, if diet and exercise were what had caused his problem, couldn't he undo the damage by going back to the way he used to eat and exercise before he lived in the Land of Plenty?

Bonny's doctor was dubious. But he gave his OK for a two-week experimental period, provided Bonny first pass a stress test to prove that his 55-year-old heart could withstand vigorous exercise.

Given only a short time to persuade his doctor that his plan could work, Bonny knew he needed to make drastic changes right away. No more sugar or processed foods. Until he got rid of his excess weight, he decided he would eat only fruit, vegetables and rice.

As for exercise, he knew he needed something strenuous that could get him the results he needed quickly. How could he get his heart pumping fast enough to scrub glucose from his blood without leaving the house while he cared for Arnold?

"I have never been in favor of using exercise equipment," he said. "It is expensive and it occupies too much space. I prefer going natural, so I thought of running the stairs – the most difficult exercise I could think of."

In the beginning, he could only climb the stairs very slowly before he would get out of breath. He broke his workouts up into small segments, but kept at it until he had accumulated two hours' worth of exercise per day.

Using the glucose meter the diabetes educator had provided him with, Bonny was stunned to see how quickly he was able to bring his blood sugar down. Within 10 days, his glucose readings were

Wed 7/24		✗	Time <46		*	Time 241		*	Time 1040		No Exercise	Time	Meals an occasional 2 hrs after a meal
			Result '37			Result 129			Result 190			Result	
Thu 7/25		*	Time 1030			Time			Time 605			Time 1134	
			Result 102			Result			Result 94			Result 98	
Fri 7/26			Time 809			Time 1141		*	Time 921			Time	
			Result 132			Result 120			Result 120			Result	
Sat 7/27			Time 940			Time 334		*	Time 1226			Time	
			Result 139			Result 131			Result 122			Result	

* 2 hrs after meal

The log book Bonny's diabetes educator gave him in 1991 show that by July 26, when he returned to see his doctor, his blood sugar readings had come down more than 300 points into the 130s and occasionally even lower.

in the 130s and at times even lower. He called the doctor, pleased to be reporting in ahead of time.

This time, Dr. Adelto Adan did not try to hand Bonny a stack of prescriptions.

"Continue doing what you are doing," he said. "These are very encouraging results."

One of Bonny's first steps in learning about his disease had been meeting with a diabetes educator who was also a dietitian. She had spent four hours teaching him to count calories and do carbohydrate exchanges using a guidebook. But as someone who was constantly studying his own habits and motivations, he knew he would be unlikely to pursue an eating program that required him to "count" his food. He preferred the idea of eating as much as he liked, providing he was only eating heart-healthy meals such as fruit, vegetables, whole grains, beans, nuts, and lean meats.

Bonny's early experiments with his glucose meter revealed that large meals, even those consisting entirely of whole foods, gave him high blood sugar readings.

"Both the doctor and the certified diabetes educator warned me that postprandial (after-eating) highs damage the body, and instructed me to avoid these highs at all costs," he said. "The trouble was, no matter how I ate, I couldn't avoid the spikes after each meal."

His solution? He quit worrying about his postprandial readings and instead focused on using his exercise to bring his blood sugar readings back down.

"When I overate, I had no choice but to correspondingly increase the amount of exercise that I must do to get the high down to a normal level," he said. "There was a time when I had a blood sugar reading of 270 mg/dl after a heavy dinner. I ran the stairs for more than 30 minutes to get it down to about 100 mg/dl."

Though Bonny's doctor didn't always agree with his methods, he couldn't argue with his results.

There was no doubt: He was off to a great start.

EMBRACING A CARB-BASED DIET

The first piece of advice most people receive about a diabetic diet is to cut carbohydrates.

And yet for the last 26 years, ever since his diagnosis in 1991, Bonny has followed a diet that is *based* on carbohydrates.

Most of his carbs come from fruit. During the summer months, when the price is right, he might go through six mangoes a day all by himself. It's not unusual for him eat an entire cantaloupe in one day. When it comes to grapes or cherries, he says, "I may finish off half a pound or even a pound in one sitting."

Bananas are among the highest-carb fruits, at 30 grams each. And yet Bonny will often consume not one but two in a single meal.

"No fruit is off limits," he says.

Bonny also eats whole grain bread, oatmeal, potatoes, rice, and vegetables, all of which contain carbohydrates. Baked goods, such as banana bread, are included in his diet so long as they are sweetened with fruits instead of sugar.

He even eats Papa John's pizza, though the type he orders has only one topping – pineapple – with no meat or cheese.

"I very well know that all type 2s have always been warned to limit their fruit and carb intake," he says. "Why did I decide at the very beginning of my life as a diabetic to eat high-carb meals? Because they are the easiest to digest.

"As they are the easiest to digest, they naturally are also the fastest to be made available to my hungry cells – especially the brain cells, which consume a lot of glucose."

As a chess aficionado who plays online chess several hours a day in addition to hosting a weekly club in his home, Bonny loves knowing his brain cells have an adequate fuel supply.

But as a type 2 diabetic, how can he get away with eating such a high-carb diet?

If you answered that he burns off excess blood sugar with vigorous exercise – not just daily but four times a day – you would be partly right.

But Bonny also attributes his ability to tolerate a diet that he estimates at nearly 70 percent carbohydrates to the fact that fruit does not activate an insulin response. Once he became aware of this, after a relative sent him a news article written by a dietitian, he began to consume all his fruit at the beginning of his meal.

The way he sees it, his pancreas is not called into action until the second course. And because in recent years he has switched to eating only two meals per day, with no snacks in between, that naturally limits how often his blood sugar is raised in the first place. (For more on how Bonny plans his meals, see "Scheduling Meals to Fight Fat" on Page 74).

Bonny's decision to focus on eating carbs was inspired by the writings of Dr. John A. McDougall, who has written extensively about the disease-prevention benefits of a whole foods, plant-based diet.

"He had a very profound influence on me," Bonny says. "What he said was very different from other articles I read about type 2 diabetes when I was newly diagnosed. He was actually the one who encouraged me to eat a lot of carbohydrates."

McDougall, who ran a clinic on a Hawaiian sugar plantation in the 1970s, has written that the basis of his dietary philosophy comes from observations he made about his patients there, many of whom came from families representing multiple generations of Asian immigrants from countries such as China, Japan, Korea, and the Philippines.

The health differences reflected over three generations in the same family, as their diets gradually shifted from rice, fruit, and vegetables to more typical Western fare, was startling, McDougall writes on his website. www.drmcdougall.com.

His elderly patients, the first-generation immigrants who still followed the rice-based diet they brought with them from their home countries, "were trim, active, and medication-free into their 90s. They had no diabetes, heart disease, arthritis, or cancers of the breast, prostate, or colon. Their children became a little fatter and sicker, and most of their grandchildren had lost all of their immunity to obesity and common diseases — in every way of appearance and health, they were full-fledged Americans."

Later, reading through medical journals, McDougall discovered that other doctors had made similar observations over the years. But another pattern emerged in his reading of these studies: Those who reverted back to their original diets erased most of their health problems.

"These pioneer scientists reported that once people stopped eating the foods that made them sick, they recovered," McDougall wrote. "They described weight loss, relief of chest pains, headaches, and arthritis. Kidney and heart failure, diabetes, and many more troubles were reversed. Volumes of research written over the previous 50 years in these library journal pages showed me how my patients could be cured with one big simple solution: a starch-based diet."

In Bonny's case, it wasn't quite that simple. Though reverting to a diet-and-exercise program more in line with what he'd been used to in the Philippines had brought his weight under control, it was clear that diet alone would not control his blood sugar. The carbohydrates in his plant-based meals, though much healthier than the highly processed carbs he had eaten before his diagnosis, did, in fact, raise his blood sugar.

But he also found that vigorous exercise – not just once a day, but multiple sessions that targeted his meals – brought his glucose readings back down.

For evidence, let's look at his readings from two dates in 2016, Jan. 17 and April 2.

On Jan. 17, a reading taken at 1:15 a.m., shortly before he went to bed, registered 108 mg/dl.

Readings taken at other points that same day – at 12:12 p.m., 6:25 p.m., and one minute after midnight (which would technically make it Jan. 18) – registered 129, 119 and 93 mg/dl, respectively.

Were there points in the day when his blood sugar went higher? Almost certainly. None of these readings were taken in the hour or two following his meals, which he typically schedules at 2 p.m. and 8 p.m.

However, if you average these four readings, spread out through the day, the resulting number is 112.25 mg/dl. While that is higher than a person who does not have diabetes would register, it falls well within the prediabetes range of 100-125.

Let's look at April 2. That day Bonny tested his blood sugar before and after his evening meal. At 7:40 p.m., before eating, it was 116 mg/dl. By 9:07 p.m., after dinner, his blood sugar was 158 mg/dl. While not dangerously high – remember, his glucose level at diagnosis was well over twice that amount – that's certainly well into problem territory.

Luckily, Bonny knew just how to take care of the problem: His usual evening exercise routine. By 1:15 a.m., after one 15-minute session of jogging up the stairs (and then carefully walking backward down the stairs to spare stress on his knees), followed by several hours of online chess, his glucose was back down to 108 mg/dl.

Because Bonny's exercise sessions invariably bring his blood sugar levels back down not too long after they go up, his hemoglobin A1C tests – which measure average blood sugar over a three-month period –- consistently fall in the normal range. (According to official medical records from the Midland Medical Center dating to 2008, the most recent available from his current doctor, his test results have ranged from a low of 5.7 percent to a high of 6.3 percent.)

Therefore he sees no reason to avoid eating the fruits he loves, or potatoes or whole grain breads, for that matter.

It should be noted that his current doctor, Dr. Gail Colby of the Mid-Michigan Medical Center in Midland, does not disapprove of his diet.

"Complex carbohydrates are preferred over simple sugars," she said. "They break down more slowly and are less likely to cause blood sugar spikes."

Bonny doesn't worry about whether his carb-based diet might be overworking his pancreas. He is skeptical when he hears so-called experts say that type 2 diabetes is a progressive disease that eventually and inevitably results in a pancreas that slows down and sometimes stops producing insulin altogether. As far as he can tell, his 81-year-old pancreas still works as well now, 26 years after his diagnosis, as it did in 1991.

"Have you heard the expression, 'use it or lose it?'" he asks. To Bonny, that doesn't just apply to his muscles but to all parts of his body, including his pancreas.

"If I don't want to lose my pancreas' ability to produce enough insulin," he reasons, "then I should keep it very, very busy by eating a lot of carbohydrates."

It may sound like a crazy idea, but it has worked for him for more than a quarter century – so long as he makes sure his heart and muscles stay just as busy as his pancreas, that is.

His longtime family physician, Dr. Adelto Adan, now retired, didn't necessarily agree with all of Bonny's ideas, but he had no objections to his unorthodox diabetic diet.

"Mr. Damocles is an example of someone who has successfully coped with his late onset Diabetes 2," Dr. Adan wrote in 2004, in a preface to a book of diabetes patients' personal stories Bonny organized called *Live Like You Have No Diabetes*.

"Mr. Damocles' recommendations are to be followed by exceptional people – people who are full of drive, inspiration and a certainty that life is worth living. Disabilities, yes, we all have some. It is up to us to be successful or to fail."

EXERCISE, THE WONDER DRUG

Given Bonny's experience in the 26 years since his diagnosis, it seems strange – almost negligent, really – that doctors don't routinely prescribe exercise as the preferred treatment option for patients with type 2 diabetes.

If such prescriptions were "used as directed," many people might find that they never required medication at all, particularly if they were willing to improve their diets in the process.

Unfortunately, not even the most informed, well intentioned doctors can guess which *type* of exercise works best for each patient. Jogging? Rollerblading? Kickboxing? Dancing? Gardening? There are literally hundreds of activities that could be considered exercise. But to be effective, the patient must take his or her "medicine" every day – preferably, multiple times a day. The doctor doesn't know which activities the patient enjoys enough to make them part of a daily routine. The trouble is, the patient likely doesn't know, either.

Given all those uncertainties, and the fact that most people never exercise as much as they intend to, it wasn't surprising that Dr. Adelto Adan followed up Bonny's diagnosis of type 2 diabetes by writing out several prescriptions.

Bonny hadn't really known what he intended to do when he begged Dr. Adan to "let me handle it my way." He had never been an athlete; chess was his game. He had never attempted an exercise program in his life.

But given just two weeks to try his experiment, Bonny put all his efforts into stair running, trying to flee diabetes with the same intensity as his family fled the invading Japanese back in Manila in December 1941.

Eventually, through much experimentation, he settled on a dosage of 60 minutes per day, broken up into four sessions of 15 minutes each.

This, it should be noted, is considerably higher than the 150 minutes of exercise per week currently recommended by the American Diabetes Association.

"Where would I be now if I followed this advice?" Bonny asks.

Bonny's do-it-yourself prescription of one hour of exercise per day – at 420 minutes per week, nearly three times the amount recommended by the ADA – has proven to be the perfect dosage for him. It is effective medication that has cost him virtually nothing. He hadn't even needed to buy a pair of workout shoes.

As for side effects, exercise may be the only "drug" that comes with positive side effects that enhance rather than detract from health. The ones Bonny experiences most often are things like improved mood, better sleep, and increased energy levels. The only "bad" side effect he has experienced is an occasional sore muscle. But this happens only rarely because he is very careful to pay attention to early signs of soreness.

Bonny estimated that he saved thousands of dollars a year by finding an alternative to the prescriptions that Dr. Adan had suggested. According to the American Diabetes Association, people with diabetes incur annual medical costs of $13,700 per year, with $7,900 of that directly attributable to diabetes. Given the skyrocketing cost of insulin in the United States over the last five years, the annual cost of diabetes has likely increased dramatically since 2012, the year of the most recent report.

"As far as I am concerned, I have been spending practically nothing," Bonny says. "The glucose meter I have been using is from Walmart, which cost me $12. The test strips I had been using were $12 for 50 strips. These Walmart products do not require me to get a doctor's prescription and they are very cheap compared to the brands usually prescribed by physicians."

Since he stopped testing his blood sugar at home in late 2016 – deciding instead to rely on his twice-yearly A1C tests unless he detects problems – Bonny's expenses have gone down even more.

Unlike his neighbor and some other people he later met on online diabetes forums, he's never experienced hypoglycemia.

He has never had to contend with the weight gain that sometimes comes from using insulin.

And most importantly, he has never had to worry about running out of his medication.

Based on Bonny's results – along with other patients who have followed in his footsteps – his current doctor has become convinced of the powerful healing properties of exercise.

Though Dr. Gail Colby of the Mid-Michigan Medical Center attributes Bonny's many years of success to his "focus and discipline," she notes that "I do have several patients who have significantly improved their lifestyle and eliminated meds and are doing well."

"I strongly encourage regular exercise," Colby says. "If you follow weight loss, exercise, and diet, you can control diabetes."

There were times over the years when Bonny could not do his stair running, due to muscle soreness or some other circumstance. But he never failed to "take his medicine." He always did *something* to raise his heart rate to the recommended levels: a formula computed by subtracting your age from the number 220, then calculating 60-80 percent of the resulting number.

For example, at the time of Bonny's diagnosis, at age 55, he would've needed to raise his heart rate to 60-80 percent of 165 (220 minus 55). That works out to between 99 and 132 beats per minute.

At his current age of 81 (as of 2017), using the same formula, he should raise his heart rate to 60-80 percent of 139, or 83 to 111 beats per minute.

Walking is perhaps the simplest way to raise your heart rate. During the years Bonny was caring for his son Arnold, however, he needed to stay in the house, near Arnold's room, in case there was trouble with the ventilator that helped him breathe.

"At home, even when it was my turn to take care of him, I could still do stair running because his ventilator would make a loud sound if he needed suctioning of his phlegm," Bonny said.

Because he didn't own any exercise equipment, and didn't wish to purchase any, on days when he couldn't run stairs he "power walked" around the house, pumping his arms and moving as briskly as possible. He would do pushups against his kitchen counter, or jog in place.

At one point, when Arnold was hospitalized about five years before he died, Bonny was forced to come up with a substitute for stair running that he could do in the hospital room. That's when he came up with a simple exercise routine he calls the Arnold Dance, a combination of squats and arm movements followed by jogging in place. (For specific instructions on this exercise, see Page 195 in the Appendix.)

"When it was my turn to care for him, my exercise had to be something that I could do without leaving his room. It is a very easy exercise that is effective in blood sugar control, can be done anywhere, anytime, and does not require any exercise equipment or special clothing."

It is also something that can be done discreetly, without attracting attention.

"The other patient in the room or the hospital people who regularly checked on Arnold never saw me dance," Bonny says. "I used the curtain to block everybody's view."

Though Bonny no longer does the specific exercise routine he calls the Arnold Dance, he performs similar movements in his "power walk" that he does around the house on days when he takes a break from his stair jogging or walking.

"During all the years that I have been enjoying the benefits I get from exercise as my only type 2 diabetes medication, I have been wondering if it will ever stop doing its good job," Bonny says. "The more I think about it, the more I am convinced that it will not.

"There is a simple way of explaining it. Any muscle movement requires fuel. A muscle that moves regularly grows stronger and bigger and requires more blood sugar for its fuel and upkeep. What used to be difficult to do gets easier as the muscle gets stronger.

"A strong and well-developed muscle constantly sends a message to the brain that it had better be kept busy for the good of the body, both physically and mentally. The more a muscle works, the more blood sugar it consumes."

It is a cycle that continually works in his favor – achieving the same or better results as prescription medications but without the expense or negative side effects.

SCHEDULING MEALS TO FIGHT FAT

Before his diagnosis, Bonny ate whatever he wanted, whenever he felt like it.

He never bothered to time his snacks so they wouldn't interfere with his meals. As far as he was concerned, anytime he was around food was snack time.

"When a poor Filipino gets the chance to come to the States, the first thing he does is eat as much as he can," he offers by way of explanation. "If he can eat every hour, he surely will. There's plenty of cheap and delicious foods here which we had never seen in the Philippines."

After his diagnosis, one of the first things Bonny did was give up snacks. Doing so would not only help him lose weight, but avoid raising his blood sugar at random intervals throughout the day.

Though it took some getting used to, going without snacks didn't necessarily mean he had to endure hunger. It just meant that he focused more closely on his meals, packing them with nutrient-dense food that filled him up.

Over time, he built a routine in which each meal was constructed with the same building blocks: a banana, a cup of grapes and a handful of unsalted nuts.

For breakfast, he would add two to four slices of raisin bread to complete his meal. For lunch and dinner, the added components were soup (typically bean, potato, mushroom, or tomato), vegetables, half a cup of rice, and lean meat. Chicken was always eaten with the skin removed. If he ate pork, the fat was always trimmed. If he was still hungry after his meal, he ate more meat or vegetables.

Bonny's enhanced meal plan, in conjunction with his exercise program, did a good job of keeping both his weight and his diabetes under control. But as he learned more about the disease, he began to incorporate new ideas into his routine.

When a relative sent him an article in which a nutritionist explained how the body was able to process the natural sugars in fruit without using insulin, for instance, he adapted his strategy and began eating fruit first at every meal. He liked the idea of his favorite foods reaching his cells quickly, without the need for an insulin boost from his pancreas.

"This must be beneficial to me because I do a lot of mental and physical activities," he reasoned. "My cells must always be adequately fed."

More recently, when he read about the benefits of intermittent fasting, Bonny decided to experiment with cutting back to two meals per day.

According to Dr. Joseph Mercola, whose mercola.com website is among those that Bonny frequents, taking a daily eating break of 14-16 hours drains glycogen reserves and forces the body into fat-burning mode. Because fat is a slow-burning energy source, Mercola writes on his website, there are fewer blood sugar highs and lows.

Recent studies, such as one published in the October 2016 *Journal of Translational Medicine*, show that several health biomarkers improved in a group of resistance trainers who practiced intermittent fasting. Besides attaining lower fat and greater muscle mass than a control group, the intermittent fasters also recorded lower blood glucose and insulin levels.

Bonny was also intrigued by an article he read about the renowned cardiologist Dr. Michael DeBakey, who died in 2007 at age 99. Though he traveled the globe, lecturing and treating world leaders such as Russian president Boris Yeltsin, DeBakey was not an indulgent diner, typically eating only one meal per day.

Did DeBakey's lone daily meal contribute to his longevity? There was no way to know. Bonny thought at some point he might try DeBakey's eating schedule. But the first step was going from three meals to two.

Bonny's meals had been scheduled at rather conventional times, with breakfast in the morning, lunch at midday and dinner in the early evening, around 7 p.m. Because he liked to stay up late and then sleep in, aiming to get eight hours of sleep between the hours of roughly 2 a.m. and 10 a.m., he moved his first meal to midday and his second meal a bit later in the evening, to around 8 p.m.

As with his adjustment to going without snacks, the move required a bit of getting used to. But before long, the sense of deprivation that came with the elimination of breakfast was quickly balanced out by the satisfaction of simplifying his routine. Now he was raising his blood sugar only twice per day instead of three times. He was spending less time preparing and cleaning up food.

Most importantly, his exercise now felt much more targeted and potent, attacking specific blood sugar spikes rather than a constant barrage of glucose overload.

Tackling his stair running each morning on an empty stomach, Bonny thought of how the lions he saw on the TV program "Wild Kingdom" waited to hunt until they felt the first pangs of hunger. Like them, he sharpened his appetite through exercise. By the time he earned his first meal of the day, he was truly able to appreciate his food.

These days Bonny's meals follow a specific format. The first course is fruit, as much of whatever he has on hand as he likes. His preference is to eat whatever is fresh and in season, which not only tastes best but tends to be the cheapest. He loves mangoes, melons, pineapple, cherries, grapes, and Golden Delicious as well as Red Delicious apples. But he will eat any kind of fruit, including berries, pears, peaches, plums, tomatoes and avocado.

After his fruit course, he eats 10 prunes to help with digestion. He may then have a chicken breast or fish, followed by a natural peanut butter sandwich made with whole-grain bread. Another option is a simple egg salad made with chopped onion and roma tomatoes, using only salt-free Mrs. Dash seasoning for extra flavor.

Vegetables of all varieties, including every type of potato and all types of beans, are fair game.

"To me, everything that comes out of the ground is either fruit or vegetable and I have no problem eating it, even if I don't know its name," he says.

Occasionally he will have a footlong roasted chicken Subway sandwich with plenty of spinach, onions and lettuce, or two slices of an extra-large

Papa John's pineapple pizza made without meat or cheese toppings.

Each meal consumed at home includes one scoop of plain nonfat Greek yogurt. He then typically finishes his meal with unsalted cashews.

"The amount depends on how full I feel," he says. "If something else has already filled me up, then I stop eating."

Bonny looks forward to his meals, but doesn't get overly hungry in the interim.

"I have always been a heavy eater," he explains. "I love food."

"But I have to schedule my eating and I always make sure that I don't overeat. By eliminating one meal, I surely reduce my food intake. If it is not my meal time, I am disciplined enough not to eat."

Some people would call that willpower. Bonny prefers to think of it as a habit that he has built through practice and repetition.

"The way I do things is generally to simplify, to make things easy to do all the time," he says. "I want to reach my 100th birthday. To succeed in reaching my goal, everything I do must keep me healthy, strong, happy, productive and feeling young."

THE THREE E'S AND DIABETES

Bonny was still in high school when he learned one of the guiding principles of his life.

There was a small space in one of the English-language newspapers devoted to meaningful quotes and words of wisdom. As a poor, shy teenager devoted to self-improvement, Bonny devoured this sort of material. He memorized quotes that appealed to him and can still recite some of them, such as "Friendship is a plant planted in my heart, and when it is always watered, it grows into love."

One item he read in the newspaper referred to "The Three E's: Economy, Effectiveness and Efficiency." He no longer remembers whom this bit of wisdom was attributed to. But from that moment on, those principles guided his actions on the chessboard as well as in life.

"Because of them, I get to be where I am now," Bonny says. Seeking the most effective, efficient and economical route to his goals helped him get a college education, secure a wife whom he continues to believe was the single best choice he ever made, and start a new life in America.

Staying focused on the Three E's helped him learn what he needed to know to start an export business that eventually made it possible for him to work at home and provide the best possible care for his son – enough so that Arnold lived more than a decade longer than the typical life expectancy of someone with Duchenne Muscular Dystrophy.

And when Bonny learned he had developed type 2 diabetes, it was the Three E's that helped him devise the simplest, cheapest, and most practical methods of managing his disease.

Some people might argue that taking medication is the simplest way to cope with diabetes, that having a pharmaceutical safety net reduces the pressure of strict adherence to a diet-and-exercise program.

However, this approach fails the Three E's test because it is not economical. In the long run, it not only becomes much more expensive but much more complicated as health problems escalate and prescriptions proliferate, along with the side effects that accompany many medications. The average patient with type 2 diabetes incurs thousands of dollars in health care costs per year.

And yet Bonny spends almost nothing on exercise, which serves as his primary diabetes medication. His stair-climbing sessions are both efficient and effective in keeping his weight and his blood sugar under control.

"My daily exercise is a very good example of how I operate," he says.

This is not to say that Bonny's exercise regimen is the one everyone should adopt. But in his case, given the need to stay home to care for Arnold, using the stairs in his home as a built-in exercise machine – requiring no added expense and raising his heart rate in the least amount of time – was the most sensible option.

Bonny typically does his exercise barefoot, which not only saves him the cost of buying athletic shoes but may also be part of the reason that his feet are so well toned and nimble for an 81-year-old. Exercise scientists believe that barefoot running can minimize injuries by strengthening the muscles and tendons in the feet. Since he began his exercise program in 1991, he has rarely experienced more than an occasional sore muscle. And yet he never takes a "rest day," believing that sticking to a routine that works so well for him is part of what keeps him happy and healthy.

"It really is not my engineering training that comes into play," he says now, reflecting on the approach that has brought him success not only in business but in defying conventional wisdom on the limitations imposed by both Arnold's disease and his own.

"It is more of the way I think. I love analyzing how things work. I don't easily believe what others think and say.

"Let's take the statement, 'Avoid high blood sugar levels as much as possible.' It is a very simple statement but the way I understand it is very different from the way others do."

Instead of fretting over how much his carb-heavy meals increased his blood sugar, Bonny focused on coming up with an exercise schedule that brought his glucose levels back within acceptable limits. The fact that his twice-yearly A1C tests never registered higher than 6.3 percent – and more importantly, the fact that he has never developed any diabetes complications such as nerve damage or heart problems – proved to him that there was no reason to fear the complex carbohydrates that made up the bulk of his meals.

In his mind, it was a classic case of the Three E's at work: Carbohydrates are not only typically cheaper than fats, dairy and animal protein, they are also easier to digest. If he could save money on fuel that provided good energy while improving his digestion and controlling his diabetes, that seemed like the most sensible alternative.

Bonny's two-meal eating schedule proved to be another Three E's success story. Eliminating one meal meant he was only raising his blood sugar twice a day. It also reduced the amount of time he spent preparing and cleaning up food. "Avoiding one meal a day is giving me more time to be more productive, healthier and have an easier time and effort to manage my diabetes."

"The Three E's are always considered in everything I do," Bonny says. "For me to have more leisure time, I have to find ways to finish my workload faster than normal."

Just as he once bought enough fast food to last his family for several meals, now he does the same with food preparation at home, cooking his heart-healthy staples in large batches to save time preparing meals later.

He stocks up on staple items when they are on sale, buying up to a year's supply of canned goods to save time as well as money.

"I easily accomplish more in less time by planning my movement," he says. "I make sure that I take the shortest route when shopping in different stores on the same day."

He even applies the Three E's principle to dining out, which he and Nemia do at least twice a week.

"In all the restaurants we go to regularly, we always do our best to make friends with the owners. We also keep the same servers. By doing so, they get to know what we want. We save time by not repeating every detail of our orders. Since our servers know us very well, it becomes easy for us to convince them to make some minor changes in their menus. We want their good and delicious food, and they want our business."

Not using diabetes medications may have saved Bonny more than $205,000 over 26 years, using the annual expense figures provided by the American Diabetes Association of $7,900 per year. (Though health care costs for diabetes were likely less in the 1990s than in 2012, when these figures were released, the costs have surely skyrocketed in the past five years along with the cost of insulin.)

He is also almost certainly healthier than he would be if he had been using drugs all this time. While it is true that he has had to work harder physically to maintain normal A1C test results, he sees other benefits from his exercise routine.

"Exercise is very effective in keeping my mind alert, in helping me have a good and sound sleep, in maintaining my weight, in keeping me healthy and strong, and in making me happy," Bonny says. "My mind does not and cannot tell me to stop exercising. From the time I found out that exercising every day is my best way to tame my type 2 diabetes, everything in me has made the decision to never stop exercising."

Following his Three E's philosophy, Bonny has gradually reduced how often he tests his blood sugar at home. In recent years he tested only a few days per year, several times per day, to get a feel for how his diet and exercise was working out.

"I save a lot of money for not using pharma drugs, for not going to the gym, for not needing nice shoes and nice clothes by exercising in our house, for eating carbohydrates – which are the cheapest foods – and for testing my blood sugar only 100 times per year," he said in a May 2016 article in Diabetes Health magazine.

In the second half of 2016 Bonny didn't perform any home finger-prick tests at all. His October A1C test result once again came back in the normal range, at 5.8 percent. Seeing that as a validation of his diet-and-exercise program, he has since decided that so long as he maintains his routine, he will no longer bother with the time and cost of home testing.

That, he notes, is a Three E's shift that is subject to change if his twice-yearly A1C test reveals any problems.

"My understanding of diet and exercise is very simple," he says. "If I take in as much as I want of healthy food, and I know how to use it so that I don't gain or lose an enormous amount of weight, then my type 2 diabetes will stay harmless."

Bonny continues to read everything he can to keep learning about diabetes, but he no longer worries about it. He has learned to trust his own instincts and experience, along with the Three E's.

"I never stop searching for new ideas, innovating and improving the things that excite me," he says.

That goes for diabetes as well as in life.

SEEING INFINITY
IN A LIMTED DIET

It may be hard for many Americans, especially those who grew up eating sugary cereals and fast food, to understand how Bonny could make such a clean break with his "Land of Plenty" diet.

If his lifelong dream was to come to the USA so that he could experience living in the Land of Plenty, then wasn't giving up sugar and convenience foods, in a sense, giving up his dream?

To understand how he could make such a sharp reversal, it may help to see the problem as a chess player would. In chess, you have to react to the situation on the gameboard and consider how the move you make at this moment will play out down the line, over the next few ensuing moves. What you absolutely cannot do is live in the past, bemoaning the loss of your bishop or some other misfortune, because doing so will not bring that game piece back and will only distract your attention from the current problem.

With this mindset, Bonny knew that continuing to eat sugar and processed foods would not only be a "bad move" in the present – resulting almost immediately in a high blood sugar reading – but would also lead to devastating losses in the future, as the buildup of excess glucose began to affect virtually every system in his body, from his eyes to the nerves in his toes.

Given the situation he found himself in after receiving his diagnosis, a mouthful of sugar no longer seemed appealing because he knew it would not lead to a good life in the Land of Plenty, but a frustrating, painful, greatly diminished life in which he could no longer enjoy himself under any circumstances.

Bonny knew he must learn to view food, like his exercise, as medicine.

Once he bought six pounds of grapes on sale for 88 cents a pound. "They looked good," he said, but he quickly discovered they were very sour. Nonetheless, by the next day he had already finished three pounds of them.

"Why do I keep eating them despite their bad taste?" he asked. "They are fruits, and fruits are good for me, sour or not. This proves that I truly eat for nutrients and not for taste."

Eating healthy food did not necessarily mean that he could no longer enjoy eating, however. Because he was eating nutritious food, and eating only at mealtimes, and burning off excess blood sugar with his exercise, he allowed himself to eat as much as he liked. For a little boy who'd once had to fill his empty stomach with water, who'd crept from his bed to open a locked cupboard with a pin so he could sneak a few handfuls of rice salvaged from the sea, it was still a glorious feeling to appreciate having a full belly. At the end of each meal, it became almost a game to add one cashew at a time until he reached the perfect point of contentment without feeling unpleasantly full.

Eliminating processed foods, at least initially, made it harder for Bonny to find sustenance in a typical American commercial zone full of convenience stores and fast food restaurants. But he quickly discovered there were still an abundance of foods he could eat.

Grocery shopping actually became easier without the distraction of bright packaging and advertising displays. Without refined sugar in his diet, he once again began to appreciate the natural sweetness in fruit. In the tropical climate of the Philippines, fruit had been plentiful and inexpensive. Now he rediscovered how good it could taste.

The produce departments in American supermarkets carried fruits and vegetables from all over the world. There were many different types of whole grains, nuts, rice, and beans. Lean meats such as fish, chicken and pork were easy to come by, generally at a very reasonable price.

Bonny discovered that he still lived in the Land of Plenty. Now he was simply more focused in how he chose to appreciate the selections available on the buffet.

He was no gourmet cook. His foods were prepared simply, as fresh as possible with little fuss. He constantly reminded himself that his food was medicine. Still, for someone who could appreciate the infinite number of ways a game of chess could play out within the limited space of a chess board, with just 16 pieces per side, the possibilities that existed within his seemingly limited diet remained limitless.

In chess, there are 400 possible positions after each player makes a single move. After two moves, that number increases to 72,084. After three moves, it goes up to 9 million. And by four moves, amazingly, the number of different possible positions is more than 288 *billion*.

The number of different scenarios that can play out in a 40-move chess game is greater than the number of electrons in the observable universe. How limited, then, is a diet in which it is almost impossible to estimate the precise number of fruits and vegetables that exist on Earth, given that there are more than 400 varieties of tomatoes alone?

Bonny is not an adventurous eater. Still, he is willing to eat any fruit or vegetable he comes across at a reasonable price. "Anything that comes out of the ground is fair game," he likes to say.

He and Nemia tend to visit the same restaurants over and over, and yet from time to time he still makes new discoveries, such as a Korean dish called Bibimbap, typically prepared with fried rice, bean sprouts, grilled chicken, spinach, carrots, zucchini, and topped with a fried egg, cooked and served in a stone bowl.

Like his exercise, Bonny never has to worry about running out of his food medicine. It is cheap and easy to stock up on staples such as rice, nuts, healthy soups, tuna, natural peanut butter, and fruit canned without added sugar.

"In this Land of Plenty, it is very easy to make big mistakes in life," Bonny says.

With so much food available, he notes, it is easy to eat thoughtlessly – to consume the wrong amounts of the wrong foods at the wrong time of day, in terms of what is best for the body.

Other "big mistakes" that are easy to make, he adds, are things like "getting lazy, stressing over petty things, having the wrong priorities, wasting time, effort, and resources on useless things, and not having enough rest time."

Though it is tempting to wish that everything was easy all the time, the reality is that challenges benefit us in ways we cannot perceive beforehand.

That has certainly been the case with Bonny, whose dietary challenges have helped improve his health much more than he ever imagined possible.

"Lucky us," Bonny says, "that we are having a very good life in the Land of Plenty."

BONNY'S 3 RULES FOR LIVING LIKE YOU HAVE NO DIABETES

In 2004, after 13 years of successfully managing his diabetes using diet and exercise as his only medicine, Bonny Damocles organized an effort by a group of people with type 2 diabetes to share what they'd learned about the most successful ways of managing their disease. This project became a book called *Live Like You Have No Diabetes*.

Not all of those who shared their stories were type 2 pioneers in the sense that term is used in this book – people who use diet and exercise as their only medication. And of course none of them truly lived as if they had no diabetes. (If Bonny did not have diabetes, he would still be eating fast food, at least on occasion. Nor would he be jogging up his stairway, unless he needed something from upstairs.)

What Bonny meant by the phrase *Live Like You Have No Diabetes* was simple: If you treat a healthy diet and regular exercise as "medicine" – working out not just once a day but multiple times, at least as often as you take in food – then your body will look and feel as if you do not have diabetes.

Bonny's self-prescribed diabetes treatment saves him thousands of dollars per year in health costs and medical bills. If everyone used his treatment method, the United States alone would save at least $245 billion a year – the total estimated economic impact of the disease, according to the American Diabetes Association, as of 2012. (That's a 41 percent increase from 2007, so one can only imagine how those projected costs have risen in the past five years.)

Though Bonny was stunned by the incredible results from his initial experiments with stair running – "I thought I hit the jackpot," he jokes now, recalling how he cut his blood sugar by more than 300 points in just 10 days – it's taken him more than a quarter century of tinkering to come up with his current diet and exercise routine.

If he could condense what he's learned into a cheat sheet – a clear set of three key guidelines to give the 1991 version of himself as he emerged from the doctor's office immediately after his diagnosis – here is what it would say:

1. You don't have to eat a low-carb diet, but you MUST stick to high-quality carbs. Do NOT eat sugar or processed foods. DO eat as many fruits and vegetables as you like, along with other natural, unprocessed plant foods such as rice, whole grains, beans, nuts, and potatoes of all kinds. These are slower burning, complex carbohydrates that provide good fuel for your body – and you are going to need good fuel, because you are no longer going to be living a sedentary life!

2. Cutting back to two meals a day, with no snacks, means you will only raise your blood sugar twice a day. This automatically makes it easier to manage your diabetes. Train yourself to eat as much healthy food as you like during each meal, so that you are full and don't feel deprived. But constantly remind yourself to not put anything else in your mouth until it is time for your second meal. Soon this will become a habit, and then you won't have to think about it anymore – it will simply become part of your usual routine.

3. Do you plan to eat more than once a day? Then you must exercise more than once a day as well. Every snack or meal will raise your blood sugar. This is nothing to worry about, provided you do some form of exercise that raises your heart rate for several minutes, enough to help clear excess glucose from your blood.

Exercise at least once before each meal and before bedtime. Choose something that is very easy to do, that does not require much preparation, cost, or favorable weather conditions. Walking around the house, moving your arms vigorously, could work. Dancing could work. Climbing your stairs could work. Simply sitting in a chair doing leg lifts and arm circles could work.

It does not matter what you do, so long as you get your heart rate up to the recommended level: Subtract your age from 220, then aim for 60-80 percent of the resulting number.

After your exercise, check your blood sugar to make sure it has returned to an acceptable level. (Note: After 25 years of demonstrating good control of your blood sugar, feel free to stop testing at home and rely on twice-yearly A1C tests to make sure no problems are developing.)

Remember: Exercise is your medicine. YOU MUST TAKE IT THREE TO FOUR TIMES A DAY OR IT WILL NOT WORK.

III. LIFE ON THE DIABETES FRONTIER

ENCOUNTERING OTHER TYPE 2 PIONEERS

Bonny was a hundred years too late to be considered an American pioneer in the classic sense of the word. By the time he and his family emigrated to America in the 1970s, Laura Ingalls Wilder's classic tales of her family's life on the frontier during the 1870s were being repackaged into the television series known as "Little House on the Prairie."

Yet when Bonny set out to tackle type 2 diabetes without medication, equipped only with diet and exercise, he was in many ways on his own, forging a path into an unknown future.

After nearly a decade of exploring on his own, he came across a couple of online communities devoted to type 2 diabetes. But Bonny was clearly very different from the others who posted there. His rejection of the conventional methods of treating the disease was viewed with suspicion and even hostility.

Bonny didn't blame the other forum members for getting irritated with him.

"It was my fault," he admits. "I was very aggressive in promoting my unusual way."

Eventually, though, after exploring several different forums, he connected with a handful of other type 2 diabetes pioneers who, like him, were attempting to control the disease using only diet and exercise.

Some, like Lyn Deal, a Georgia woman who had been diagnosed in 2000 at age 52, had the support of their doctors. Others, such as Susanne Rice, a Vermont woman who had been diagnosed at age

39, did not. After a few weeks of experimenting with her diet took her fasting blood glucose from 350 to 150, Susanne informed her doctor she wasn't ready to start the medications she recommended.

"This upset her," Rice wrote in her contribution to Bonny's 2004 book of personal stories about diabetes called *Live Like You Have No Diabetes*. "But we agreed that if my next A1C was down in a few weeks, she would agree to let me go with diet and exercise."

Eight weeks later, Rice's A1C registered 6.3 percent, down from a dangerously high 14+ at diagnosis. Over the next few years her test results varied from 4.9 to 5.3 percent, all well within the normal range.

One of the type 2 diabetics Bonny met online said she was determined to manage her disease with diet and exercise because that's what her mother had done – and lived to age 93 with no complications.

"Hard work was her exercise, and it paid off," wrote Marie Rainey, who recalled that her mother likely had diabetes for at least 30 years. Though she initially changed her diet and lost a great deal of weight early on, over time she went back to traditional farm foods. Her active lifestyle as a "hard-working farm lady" was likely what made all the difference. Marie noted that her mom painted the exterior of the family's farmhouse while in her 80s, and was still mowing the lawn and trimming weeds up until she fell and broke her hip at age 93.

"She loved being busy and actually created work for herself," Marie wrote. "My mother's story proves that hard work and lots of physical exercise go a long way in controlling diabetes."

Though Bonny never met Marie's mother or saw any documentation of her long-term success in managing diabetes without medication, he was inspired by Marie's stories about the hard-working Texas farm lady. They reminded him of another old-timer he'd heard about from a classmate at his engineering school in the Philippines.

Bonny's friend described how his father managed to control his Type 2 diabetes without drugs for many years because he walked several miles twice a day going to and from work.

"From their stories, nothing was mentioned about their food intake," Bonny noted. "It would then appear to me that all that they needed was plenty of physical activities."

Maybe so. But unlike these old-timers from another generation, seemingly legendary figures whose stories provided inspiration but not much in the way of details, neither Bonny nor the type 2 diabetics he met online had hard physical labor automatically wired into their lives. All of them had to make special arrangements to put their bodies through a workout.

"There is one big difference in my mother and myself, a big difference," wrote Marie. "She was a hard-working farm lady all her life, and I am a sedentary city gal."

In addition to type 2 diabetes, Marie had many other problems that her mother never had to contend with, including fibromyalgia, irritable bowel syndrome, carpal tunnel syndrome, and a breathing difficulty her doctors called carbon dioxide deficiency. Exercise was a struggle, as Marie's legs were weak and her breathing labored. But she worked hard at figuring out a diet that kept her blood sugar in check and worked just as hard at staying positive, another key coping mechanism she attributed to her mother.

"I believe controlling diabetes without medication as long as possible will be better for my body in the long run," she wrote in 2004.

Though exercise became increasingly difficult for Marie over the years, she has kept up her positive attitude. Now 82 years old, as of 2017, she continues to control her diabetes without medication. After more than 17 years of carefully watching her diet, she says she has a pretty good idea what makes her blood sugar go up, and does her best to avoid those foods.

"The problem with many diabetics is, they do not want to give up or limit what they like to eat or how much," she says. "They prefer to pop pills and eat what they want."

BUILDING MENTAL TOUGHNESS TO LOSE WEIGHT

It might seem that Bonny has a built-in advantage when it comes to willpower because he knows what it feels like to go several days without food. Being able to tap the built-in memories of a child who endured starvation during the Japanese occupation of the Philippines during World War II puts every other dietary adjustment in perspective.

"Mental toughness is actually a natural part of me," Bonny says. "I keep on telling people that I don't get hungry very easily because of my experience during my childhood when we had nothing to eat for several days in a row."

Bonny became a hearty eater in adulthood. Forcing himself to eat only at scheduled mealtimes may have been somewhat of a hardship when he initially made the adjustment after his diagnosis. But that is nothing compared with the satisfaction he feels in knowing that he can eat as much as he likes during his meals, so long as he sticks to unprocessed, heart-healthy foods.

Studies show that people who undergo adversity often develop coping skills that help them deal with other problems that crop up in life. It's like the old saying, "What doesn't kill you makes you stronger." Researchers call this psychological resilience.

In sports, coaches refer to a similar quality in athletes who have learned from past challenges as "mental toughness." In dieting, this type of focus and determination to overcome obstacles is often referred to as willpower.

But no matter what you call it, it's a skill that can be developed, like a muscle that gets stronger with practice. The key is to search within yourself for times in the past when you have been successful in overcoming a challenge.

For many people who developed type 1 diabetes in their youth, it is the disease itself that they credit with building their mental toughness. Tom Higham, executive director of FutureEverything, one of the United Kingdom's leading festivals in digital art and innovation, has said that his determination to compete in sports as a youth despite having type 1 diabetes gave him an edge in other aspects of his life.

"I think that a chronic condition can bring perspective that can help you to focus on what you want, and what it is that matters to you," Higham said in a June 29, 2015 post on JDRF.org, the site of the Juvenile Diabetes Research Foundation. "Conditions like this are hard, they are relentless, but they build a discipline and a toughness that is hard to find otherwise."

Type 2 diabetes is very different from Type 1 diabetes. It impacts the body much differently, and it typically doesn't occur until middle age – long after lifestyle habits and personality traits have been established. By the time they develop type 2 diabetes, many people are woefully out of shape and have already experienced decades of futility at managing their weight. No matter how successful they may feel in their professional lives, they may feel helpless when it comes to improving their health.

And yet it can be done. Just ask Phillip Brenneman, whom co-author Tanya Isch Caylor interviewed for a January 2017 article at diabeteshealth.com.

Brenneman was in his mid-40s when he realized he had to do a better job of managing his type 2 diabetes or he might not live to see his daughter, then age 4, grow up. At 400 pounds, he lacked the mobility to attempt any kind of traditional exercise program. But Brenneman knew he was only a few years away from the age his mother was when she died of complications from type 2 diabetes. In February 2015, the morning after a gluttonous Super Bowl party, the Garrett, Ind., man decided he needed to quit worrying and do something about his health problems.

Because his challenge was so intimidating, Brenneman focused on taking it one step at a time. He had never had success with dieting, so he didn't go on a diet. He simply made changes to what he had been doing previously. Instead of picking up fast food on the way home from work, he stopped at the grocery store and bought healthy food to cook at home. As for exercise, all he could manage initially were simple arm circles and leg lifts while sitting in a chair.

It wasn't much. But those changes helped him lose a few pounds, which encouraged him to try new things. He joined his local YMCA. He packed his lunch so he would always know ahead of time what he was going to eat.

Eventually Brenneman lost 200 pounds simply by focusing on one step at a time, studying the Internet for nutrition and exercise tips that he implemented into his routine.

"Most people know what they're doing wrong," said Brenneman, who no longer needs Metformin and insulin to control his diabetes. "You've got to own up to it. I'm the one who put all that unhealthy stuff in my body."

The path to developing mental toughness is different for everyone, because it's a journey built on personal experience. Yet the first step is almost always the same: Stop feeling sorry for yourself and focus on tangible steps that can improve the situation.

When Tom Ross, one of the type 2 pioneers Bonny met through an online forum, received a phone message in 2001 informing him his lab tests indicated he had developed type 2 diabetes, he was mortified. His doctor had been warning him for years that something like this could happen if he didn't lose weight and get in shape. On his blog, notmedicatedyet.com, Ross wrote that he dreaded the humiliation of his upcoming doctor's appointment almost more than he dreaded the disease itself.

"Then it dawned on me that I might be able to regain my dignity if I first regained the initiative," he wrote.

Ross decided to educate himself about diabetes and start a diet and exercise program without waiting for his doctor's advice. Even if his doctor told him what he was doing was wrong, he figured, it would be good to show that he was at least doing *something*.

"Instead of waiting nervously for him to tell me what to do," Ross wrote, "I would explain to him what I was already doing, and see what he thought of it."

Ross' plan worked. His doctor approved of his workout plan and his low-fat vegetarian diet. Within six months he lost 50 pounds and his lab tests had returned to normal, all without resorting to any diabetes medications.

And it all started by deciding to act instead of feeling hopeless and helpless.

"When I say that improvement is possible, I don't mean that it happens to certain lucky people, and you should sit around waiting to see whether or not it is going to happen to you," Ross wrote on his blog. "Trust me: if you sit around waiting, it *isn't* going to happen to you. The kind of improvement I'm talking about is possible in the sense that it can happen if you choose to make it happen. The probability that it will just happen by itself is, unfortunately, zero."

Though none of the other type 2 pioneers Bonny has encountered over the years has had to endure the sort of challenges he faced growing up in the Philippines during World War II, most were able to reach deep inside themselves to find the courage to fight their disease.

In some cases, it helped knowing they were not alone in their struggles, that there were other people who were fighting similar battles. However, in the end, to have true success, taking personal responsibility is important.

"Do not expect your doctor to control this disease for you," wrote Bonny's fellow type 2 pioneer Susanne Rice in *Live Like You Have No Diabetes*. "This is YOUR disease. Own it, learn about it, discover what it does to your body and what will manage it."

And if your doctor isn't supportive, she added, "fire him (or her) and get another."

By the time Bonny developed type 2 diabetes, he had decades of experience watching and questioning others to see what he could learn. What mistakes did he and others make that he could learn from? What did other people who were more successful do differently? Searching for the answers to those questions helped him take a more successful path through life.

It also helped him form a successful coping strategy when he developed diabetes.

"Unless a person learns to be curious, I think that he won't go far," Bonny says. "I doubt very much if I can teach others to be disciplined and mentally tough. The only thing I may be able to do is inspire them.

"They should find for themselves the answers to the question, 'What is behind someone's success?' "

MORE TIPS FROM THE TYPE 2 TRADING POST

The other type 2 diabetes pioneers Bonny met online were a diverse group, and not just geographically. Whatever trials they faced in their own unique diabetes adventures, they knew they could find what they needed at their favorite forums: Not just news and information that they were unlikely to hear anywhere else, but a resupply of motivation and courage to keep going.

Without the support she'd found online, wrote a Missouri woman named Shelly Sparks, "I doubt I would've had the fortitude to face what I have in the past two years."

Though they were united in their belief that the secret to living well with diabetes was using diet and exercise rather than medication, they all had their own unique ways of doing things.

Pam Chapin of Washington State was convinced that herbs and natural supplements were critical to her success and was always sharing her recommendations with others. Cravings for specific foods, she warned, could be a sign that the body was depleted in certain nutrients.

"For example, if you've just got to have your chocolate fix, you may be depleted in magnesium," she wrote. "If you crave carbs and sugars, you may be depleted in chromium."

Marie Rainey, Bonny's friend from Texas, kept herself from eating certain troublesome foods by imagining "an invisible zipper" across her mouth.

"Just imagining that closed zipper has helped me avoid nibbling," she wrote. "Try it. It works!"

Many had harrowing health misadventures in their past – close calls and tales of triumph over seemingly insurmountable odds.

A Texas woman named Judie Garner was repeatedly rushed to the emergency room over a two-year period with dangerously high blood pressure, a pounding heart and a beet-red face. Doctors couldn't say what was causing these episodes. Test results invariably came back inconclusive, including a fasting blood glucose test that invariably registered around 90 points – not even high enough to be considered in the prediabetic range.

"On one hospital visit, a nurse told me that my heart was not going to take much more," Garner wrote. "That really scared me, since they could never find out what was wrong."

Finally, after yet another episode that generated not only a red face but blisters on Garner's cheeks, a new doctor ordered an A1C test. It revealed that despite the apparently normal result on her fasting blood glucose tests, she did in fact have type 2 diabetes.

Garner was afraid to take the medications the doctor prescribed because she had several drug allergies. She asked if she could try diet and exercise instead. Her doctor agreed, but warned that she would have to work extremely hard to achieve results.

The first thing she did when she got home was find an online diabetes forum for information and support. Then she wasted no time setting up a diet-and-exercise program that she followed zealously, fearful of what would happen if she failed.

"When I went back for my three-month check, the doctor was shocked," she wrote. "I had lost 42 pounds and all my symptoms were gone. I felt so good!"

Though they were united in their belief that the secret to living well with diabetes was rejecting drugs in favor of diet and exercise, many type 2 pioneers reported strange incidents that showed just how varied individual responses could be.

While traveling, Marie Rainey discovered that she could get away with eating more carbohydrates, including spaghetti and cookies, at higher altitudes. Her theory was that it had something to do with her lungs having to work harder to breathe, even when she wasn't exercising.

But a trip the following year seemed to cancel out her earlier findings.

"Never take for granted that what works one time will work another time!" she wrote, noting that on the second trip a pasta dinner "cost me six miles on the treadmill."

Shelly Sparks reported that stress made it harder for her to control her blood sugar even when she was exercising. Half an hour of meditation, on the other hand, could lower her blood sugar by up to 30 points with no exercise at all.

The most effective combination, she reported, seemed to be the incongruous pairing of relaxing music with vigorous exercise.

Still, she noted, "a diabetic must be relentlessly flexible because the body changes. It ebbs and flows like the tide, and we have to be able to meet the challenges that are always around the corner."

THE TRUTH ABOUT REVERSING DIABETES

In recent years, stories of people who have successfully "reversed" their diabetes have popped up in the news from time to time.

Actor Drew Carey lost 80 pounds in 2010 and got off his diabetes medications, leading him to tell *People* magazine, "I'm not diabetic anymore. No medication required."

In 2016 actor Tom Hanks revealed that he had been diagnosed with type 2 diabetes, but said his doctor told him he could get rid of the disease with weight loss and exercise.

That August, reality TV star Rob Kardashian told *People* magazine that losing weight had helped him "become diabetes-free."

Can type 2 diabetes really be reversed? If so, what does that really mean?

Research increasingly shows what Bonny and other type 2 diabetes pioneers have known for years – that for many people, diet and exercise can bring blood sugar readings down to normal or nearly normal levels. In a 2014 study published in the *Journal of the American Medical Association*, simply receiving regular counseling on diet and exercise helped 11.5 percent of obese adults diagnosed with type 2 diabetes to bring their blood sugar levels down without medication.

Dr. Joel Fuhrman, author of *The End of Diabetes*, claims that he has helped many of his patients get off diabetes medications by switching to a nutrient-dense diet consisting primarily of whole plant foods. In a case study published in 2012 in the *Open Journal of Preventative Medicine*, Fuhrman and fellow researchers reported that 90 percent of participants with type 2 diabetes were able to eliminate or at least reduce their medications. The average A1C test result for patients in the study dropped from 8.2 to 5.8 percent, taking it down into the normal range.

But true diabetes pioneers know that "reversing" diabetes isn't the same as "curing" diabetes. Just because your blood sugar levels have returned to normal or prediabetes levels doesn't mean you can go back to the same kind of life you were living prior to diagnosis.

Just ask Rob Kardashian, who was back in the pages of *People* magazine at the end of 2016 after having been rushed to the hospital for a "diabetes-related episode." The reason? He had reverted to "a terrible diet," apparently because of depression related to his love life.

The other type 2 pioneers Bonny got to know through various online diabetes forums knew that if they went back to the lifestyle that had made them sick in the first place, they would suffer serious consequences.

"I work out an hour a day, five days a week, minimum," wrote Susanne Rice, one of the people who contributed her story to *Live Like You Have No Diabetes*. "If I stop, the levels creep up and I will be in trouble. I HAVE to exercise. It is required for my body or I will have to have medication in its place."

Rice said she often thinks of diabetes as a sleeping dog.

"Take care of it and it will lie there peacefully and you can nearly forget it's there," she wrote. "Forget to tend it, and it will rear its ugly head."

Another type 2 pioneer Bonny met through an online forum, Tom Ross, said that weight loss and regular exercise helped him control his blood sugar so well that after two years, his doctor informed him he was no longer considered a diabetes patient.

But Ross, a technical writer from California who later began blogging about his diabetes experiences at notmedicatedyet.com, said he wanted to emphasize that he was not suggesting that diabetes is curable. What his doctor meant, he wrote in a blog post, is that he had demonstrated he was capable of consistently controlling his blood sugar without medication.

"But let me be realistic here," Ross wrote. "The only reason my blood sugar level stays normal is that I work hard at keeping it that way."

Ross said he noticed that if he slacks off his running and cycling workouts due to illness or injury – or if his exercise doesn't keep pace with his eating, such as sometimes happens during the holidays – then his blood sugar levels edge higher.

"The change is not large or sudden, but there is no mistaking the trend," he wrote. "I estimate that, if I should ever let my guard down and go back to living the way I once did, my blood sugar would probably climb back up to diabetic levels within three weeks."

From the very beginning, Bonny took the idea of reversing diabetes literally. When he received his diabetes diagnosis in 1991, he set out to undo the damage his unhealthy lifestyle had caused by essentially doing the opposite of what had caused the problem.

"I reached the conclusion that I became diabetic because I stopped eating fruits, vegetables, rice, and fish, and I became very lazy physically," he wrote in *Live Like You Have No Diabetes*. "I also realized that there was only one way for me to get back to my health: Go back to what I used to eat and what I used to do physically."

Instead of the high-calorie, high-sugar convenience food he'd gotten used to, Bonny went back to eating mostly plant foods supplemented with a small amount of lean meat. He couldn't go back to walking everywhere the way he used to do in the Philippines, because he worked from home and had to care for his son. But he did the next best thing, by scheduling multiple exercise sessions each day, jogging up and down the stairs in his home.

One day, after more than three years of being a model "reformed" diabetes patient, a friend suggested to him that he must be cured.

Bonny wanted to believe him.

"So I drastically reduced my stair-running time to practically none on some days and started eating the wrong foods for me: steaks, fried chicken, pork chops, and other high fat foods."

Then one day, out of curiosity, he tested his blood sugar.

"It was 486 mg/dl. I nearly fainted."

Though Bonny has modified his exercise regimen in the years since, doing only as much as he needs to keep his blood sugar in check and switching to walking instead of running for safety purposes, he knows better than to let up.

"I know, as all type 2 diabetics know, that once a diabetic, always a diabetic. I will never get rid of this disease."

Bonny has no expectation that he might someday be cured, either through his own efforts or some miraculous new drug that may come along. But he is a big believer in *reversing* diabetes – providing people are disciplined enough to stay in that "reverse" gear.

"Type 2 diabetes is actually an easy disease to manage," he says. "All it takes is for a type 2 diabetic to realize that its cause or causes should be reversed."

Moving along in reverse mode may not come naturally to everyone. But Bonny wholeheartedly believes that the rewards – "a good, healthy, and happy life" – are well worth it.

OLDEST LIVING TYPE 2 PIONEER?

As the years passed and Bonny got to know more people through visiting online diabetes forums, he began to wonder if anyone else with type 2 diabetes had ever gone 25 years without resorting to drugs.

He knew that his friend Marie Rainey believed her mother, a "hard-working Texas farm lady," had lived with type 2 diabetes for at least that long without using medication. But Marie's mother had died in 2003, and Bonny did not know if the details of her case had ever been officially documented.

The Joslin Center for Diabetes awards medals to people with type 1 diabetes who reach longevity milestones of 50 years or more. People who have type 1 diabetes, which most often strikes people in childhood or their teen years, cannot make sufficient amounts of insulin. Before insulin was developed in the 1920s, they were basically doomed to die by middle age, if not sooner. The development of insulin injections and, later on, insulin pumps that have grown increasingly sophisticated, have dramatically increased the lifespans of type 1 diabetes patients. Now it is not unusual for people to live 75 years or more after diagnosis.

Since 1996, the Joslin Center has awarded 75-year medals to 28 people with type 1 diabetes. In 2013, the center awarded its first 80-year medal to a Fayetteville, N.Y., man named Spencer Wallace, who was then 89 years old. Given the number of centenarians alive today, and the fact that type 1 diabetes is sometimes diagnosed in the first few years of life, it is not unthinkable that someday the Joslin Center will award a century medal to someone.

But the Joslin Center does not maintain longevity records for people with type 2 diabetes, and no other agency appears to do so, either. Perhaps this is because the majority of people who develop type 2 diabetes do so after they've already lived half a century or more. It's not unusual for people with type 2 diabetes to live into their 80s. The trouble is, most elderly type 2 diabetes patients have not only been taking multiple medications for many years, but have also been suffering from increasingly debilitating complications for several years as well.

Bonny was 55 when he was diagnosed. Now 81, he has yet to find anyone who has gone 25 years or more successfully managing type 2 diabetes without drugs.

David Mendosa, a journalist and diabetes advocate who maintains the website mendosa.com, was diagnosed with diabetes in 1994, three years after Bonny. Through his many books, articles and blog posts Mendosa may have done more to help educate others about this disease than anyone who isn't a scientist or a doctor.

"Diabetes is a disease that perhaps more than any other depends much more on the patient than on the doctor," Mendosa writes on his website.

In a May 29, 2016 e-mail, Mendosa told Bonny that he knew of no one who had topped Bonny's apparent longevity record for type 2 diabetes with no drugs and no complications.

Though Mendosa said he was now maintaining a healthy weight of 156 pounds – literally half the 312 pounds he weighed at his heaviest – he has not always been drug-free. In 2007, he relied on a new drug called Byetta that he credits with changing his life. Though he had previously brought his blood sugar under control, it was during this time that he finally lost a significant amount of weight. He was extremely pleased with his experience using that drug, a GLP-1 agonist, and he went on to write a book about it.

"Still, I wanted to manage my diabetes without any drugs at all," Mendosa said in a Dec. 8, 2012 interview on healthcentral.com.

By January 2017, Mendosa had been drug-free for several years and considered his diabetes to be in remission, with monthly A1C tests that averaged just above 5 percent. Unlike Bonny, he followed a strict low-carb diet because that approach seemed to work best for him.

"I did get some complications of diabetes before I lost a lot of weight and started following a very low carb diet," Mendosa told Bonny in a Jan. 2, 2017 email. "But I reversed all of the complications and am healthier now than I have ever been – even though I am 81 years old!"

Unfortunately, just a short time later Mendosa was diagnosed with liver cancer. He died on May 8, 2017. In his final blog post, just a few days before his death, he wrote, "I am glad to be able to write that this type of cancer is not one of the many complications of diabetes."

Blondie Fram, one of the few type 2 diabetics featured in Dr. Sheri R. Colberg's 2007 book, *50 Secrets of the Longest Living People with Diabetes*, was credited with "living well with type 2 diabetes for at least four decades" before her death in 2008 at age 93.

Fram initially controlled her diabetes with diet and exercise alone before she was put on insulin by her son-in-law, Dr. Aaron Vinik, a prominent neuropathy specialist at Strelitz Diabetes Center in Norfolk, Va. Though Fram lived an active, engaged and ultimately long life, she injected insulin for decades, according to her daughter,

Etta Vinik, associate director of education at the Strelitz Center.

In a May 2016 email, Colberg said she knew of no one with type 2 diabetes who has gone longer than Bonny has with neither drugs nor complications.

But "it is possible, especially with lots of regular physical activity," Colberg wrote in a separate email. "Type 2 diabetes involves insulin resistance, and much of that resistance stems from not having appropriate room to store carbohydrates in muscles as glycogen. When people exercise regularly (particularly doing harder workouts), they use up muscle glycogen, which leaves room for the body to handle more carbs when they eat them."

In March 2017, Bonny submitted an application to the Guinness Book of World Records, to see if his entry in a new category – "Longest time as a healthy drug-free type 2 diabetic" – would be accepted.

As of the publication of this book, his application is still under review.

If his case is accepted and verified, however, it would not be the first diabetes entry included in the Guinness Book of World Records.

The world record for the highest blood glucose level was set by a 6-year-old boy named Michael Patrick Buonocore on March 23, 2008, when he was admitted to an emergency room at a hospital in East Stroudsburg, Pa., with a reading of 2,656 mg/dL. Buonocore, who was diagnosed with type 1 diabetes, recovered.

In 2014, another type 1 diabetes patient set a world record, though 33-year-old Alex Collins' feat had nothing to do with his blood sugar.

Collins, who was diagnosed the previous year, set the record for "fastest marathon dressed in an animal costume" when he finished the London Marathon in 2 hours, 48 minutes while wearing a full-body tiger suit.

IV. LESSONS LEARNED OVER THE YEARS

TALK TO YOUR DOCTOR –
BUT LISTEN TO YOUR BODY

One day, after many years of living with diabetes, Bonny ran into the doctor who had diagnosed him. Dr. Adelto Adan had served as his longtime family physician but had since retired.

Now that they were no longer doctor and patient, Bonny could not resist asking Dr. Adan why he had allowed Bonny to hold off on taking the prescription he had written out for diabetes medication.

"I always believe that my patients know their bodies better than I do," Dr. Adan told him. "As a physician, I ask my patients probing questions for me to know what really ails them and then I prescribe what I think is the appropriate medication. If a patient suggests a better prescription, I give in and see what happens. After a few days, the patient and I find out the actual outcome of our mutual decision, and it usually is good."

The more Bonny experimented with his diabetes-management techniques over the years, the more interested he became in taking charge of other aspects of his health as well.

"I had been taking blood pressure medication long before we came to the U.S.," he said. "Most Filipinos have blood pressure problems because of the salty foods we have been eating. We have salted eggs, salted fish, and salted most everything. In short, salt is the material used for preserving food in the Philippines. I thought that I had to be on blood pressure medication forever."

In 2013, he read a medical report suggesting that the new upper limit for blood pressure in senior citizens should be updated from 120/90 to 150/90. Because his readings fell within that range, he decided to experiment with trying to control his blood pressure with dark cocoa powder, which was a suggestion he read in another medical report online.

"I stopped taking my low-dose blood pressure medication in December. In April of the following year, I told our family physician what I had done. My blood pressure reading in her office was something like 140/88. She gave me her approval, but I had to make sure that the systolic reading should go no higher than 160. From then up to now, my blood pressure has been within the new limits," Bonny reported in the fall of 2016.

Tracking his body's responses in regard to other issues, Bonny discovered that shrimp and beef caused flare-ups of gout. Avoiding those foods kept that problem in check.

Experimenting with his fluid intake, he discovered the ideal amount that kept his enlarged prostate (typical for a man his age) from awakening him at night with the urge to make a trip to the bathroom.

"For quite some time now I have been drinking between 50 ounces and 55 ounces of water every day," he reports. "My last drink must be no later than 7:30 p.m. for me to avoid getting up several times during the night" after going to bed around 1 a.m.

"Am I taking much less fluid than the healthy amount? No, because all the fruits and vegetables that I eat every day are more than 75 percent water."

With all of his health experiments, Bonny continues to monitor the situation to look for changes that may indicate a need to adjust his methods.

In early 2017, when his daily blood pressure readings began to creep up despite putting liberal amounts of cocoa powder in his oatmeal or banana bread, he decided to go back on his low-dose blood pressure medication.

Around the same time, after more than 25 years of avoiding foods with sugar, he decided to allow himself an occasional serving of his wife's sweet rice pudding, a Filipino dessert known as Biko. (This dish is made with glutinous rice, which is also known as sticky rice, or "malagkit" in the Tagalog or Filipino language. Nemia's recipe can be found in the Appendix.)

"After reaching my 25th year as a type 2, and now that I am 81 years old, I am getting bold," he said. "So far so good. I have not felt anything going bad yet. My eyesight is still the same and I am not losing any feelings yet in my toes.

"You know me, I am always experimenting."

DINING OUT
AND SPECIAL OCCASIONS

Some people can successfully monitor their diet, but then fall apart when dining in a restaurant or when the holidays or some other special occasion comes up. The trouble is, just about anything can be considered a special occasion. It is hard to decline when a co-worker brings a birthday treat into the office, or to be disciplined about your diet when a friend invites you to lunch or there's a potluck meal at your church.

Bonny doesn't avoid restaurants. In fact, he likes to joke that he has a "bad habit of inviting everybody I meet" to lunch. He and Nemia go out to eat at least twice a week, just the two of them, in addition to meeting other people for restaurant meals.

"We used to take out the whole staff of our First United Methodist Church of Midland every year to Genji's, a Japanese Restaurant," Bonny says. Now they have lunch there with four different members of the church every 45 days. They even take their mailman out to lunch at Olive Garden three or four times a year.

Bonny acknowledges he has less control over what goes into his food at a restaurant. Though he never knowingly orders anything with sugar, salt or artificial ingredients, he admits there may be times when there is salt or sugar lurking in bread, soup or salad dressings, particularly if they are dining at a chain restaurant such as Applebee's or Panera Bread.

But he and Nemia's habit of dining at familiar establishments, whether locally owned or franchised, makes it much easier to find out what goes into the food prepared in the restaurant's kitchen. And in general, it makes eating decisions much easier. They almost always know in advance what's on the menu. And since they know the servers, it is not only easier to make special requests, it often is not even necessary. Usually the person taking their order already knows how they like certain dishes prepared.

At a favorite local restaurant called Asian Express, for instance, Bonny recently tried a Korean dish called Bibimbap. It is typically prepared with fried rice, bean sprouts, grilled chicken, spinach, carrots, zucchini, and topped with a fried egg, all cooked and served in the same stone bowl. Bonny liked the dish very much, but the second time he ordered it he requested that the carrots and zucchini be replaced with extra spinach and bean sprouts. Now that his regular server knows this, he doesn't even to have to ask. She also knows he likes his food prepared with no salt or MSG, while Nemia prefers her dishes to be low sodium but not completely devoid of salt.

What if you follow a certain meal schedule that gets disrupted when someone invites you out to eat?

Bonny and Nemia both converted to eating only two meals a day several years ago, but they eat at different times. Bonny, who typically doesn't go to bed until 1 or 2 a.m. after a few hours of playing online chess, usually sleeps until 10 a.m.

He eats his first meal between noon and 1 p.m. and his second meal between 8 and 9 p.m. Nemia, who also stays up late but naps in the afternoon, rises earlier. She eats her first meal between 7 and 8 a.m. and her second meal between 2 and 3 p.m.

When they go out to eat on Wednesdays and Saturdays, their favorite time to dine is 2 p.m. This way the lunch crowd has dissipated. There is less noise, less distraction for their server and less chance of being exposed to sick people.

Nemia doesn't have to make any adjustment at all, because 2 p.m. is her usual dining time at home as well.

"What Nemia wants, Nemia gets," Bonny says. "It was my promise to her when I begged her to marry me."

He is teasing, but only a little. He is a big believer in the saying, "Happy wife, happy life." It is not necessarily something he read in that little corner of the newspaper in Manila growing up, where he learned of the Three E's. But paying close attention to his wife's happiness in their nearly 60 years together has always worked out well for him.

In reality, though, he admits dining slightly later than his usual mealtime is not a difficult adjustment to make. He simply eats his fruit and yogurt at home before they leave, then consumes his meat and vegetables at the restaurant, along with any soup, salad or bread he may order that day.

As for celebrations, Bonny learned a long time ago to separate the joy he feels on such occasions from the food he consumes. (Feasting is not an issue for him because he always eats as much good healthy food as he likes without making himself feel miserable.)

When Bonny and Nemia host Christmas or Thanksgiving meals, they pay for the food but ask their daughter, Arlene, and other friends and relatives to bring all the typical American dishes they like.

"Doing things this way makes it very easy, convenient, simple for us and good for all party attendees because everything is their choice, home-cooked, and all leftovers leave with them," Bonny explains.

In 2016, the Thanksgiving meal served at Bonny and Nemia's home included two turkeys, one spiral ham, four bottles of wine, cakes "and all the other things that go with turkeys and ham."

Bonny was just finishing his first meal of the day when some of the guests arrived. He explained what he was eating and why. Shortly afterward, when the holiday meal was set out, "the ham was salty so I did not dare taste it," he said. "The two turkeys looked good so I tried a big piece of the white meat, which was unsalted. It was delicious."

Celebrations are plentiful in the Philippines. Throughout the year, each town in the country has its annual fiesta, a time "when anybody can go in somebody's home and join the family in the celebration of the town's patron saint." The Christmas season stretches from Nov. 2, the day after All Saints Day, to Jan. 6, traditionally known as Three Kings Day.

"I think that the Philippines is the only country that celebrates nearly every day," Bonny says. He likes to say that he and Nemia celebrate every day as well. "Why do I say that I celebrate every day? Because of what I learned from my Motherland."

But Bonny and Nemia's way of celebrating does not involve decorations, feasting or drinking. In fact, Bonny has never been a drinker or a smoker, noting that his only "bad habit" is staying up late playing online chess. They celebrate in simple ways, such as by wishing each other Happy Birthday every time they see the numbers 12 or 16, representing the days of the month they were each born.

"Lately, we added the numbers 36 and 37," representing the years they were born. "So there are now four numbers which will make us greet each other happy birthday," he explains.

They also celebrate well-timed stock market decisions, the arrival of a newly leased car, even simple things like an unexpected good buy on natural peanut butter at Kroger.

"To us, celebration is anything extraordinary that we do for ourselves and are grateful for it," he explains.

On their daily visits to Arnold's grave, Bonny pats the top of his tombstone and wishes him "Happy New Year, Happy Birthday, Merry Christmas," going through a list of every possible fond greeting he can think of for his youngest son. In many ways, he and Nemia like to think he has become their guardian angel who watches over them.

There is always a story involved with a guardian angel or, in the case of the fiestas celebrated in Philippine villages, a patron saint. In Arnold's case, the narrative Bonny and Nemia have woven together over the years has to do with a movie, a TV program, and a doorbell.

The movie is the 1990 film "Ghost," starring Patrick Swayze.

"At the very start of the story, Patrick died in an accident. He had a girlfriend whom he loved very much. Through his spirit, he always warned his girlfriend of impending dangers. Arnold and I watched this movie on TV several times. It really was a very fascinating story.

"There was another TV presentation that Arnold and I loved watching. It was about a scientist trying to figure out a way to communicate with dead people. In one segment, he had a proposition that two people should come up with an idea for one of them to send signals to the living person after he dies."

Bonny and Arnold never came up with such a signal before Arnold's death in 1999. But a few years afterward, Bonny bought a GE wireless doorbell with several different chimes. He ultimately decided the doorbell was impractical and never installed it. Because it could also be used as a clock, however, he set it in their master bathroom.

Somedays the clock is silent. Other days, it chimes at unexpected times. The strange thing is that this almost always seems to happen when Bonny and Nemia are discussing something they are happy or excited about.

"I told this story to some relatives and friends. One smart one said that any electrical device in the vicinity could be the trigger of the chime," Bonny said.

But one day, during a period of time when they had no electricity for three days, he wished that the doorbell clock would ring – and it did.

"Calling Arnold our Guardian Angel is begging him to be one, like Patrick Swayze in the movie 'Ghost,'" Bonny says.

Hearing the doorbell ring is one of their favorite celebrations of all. And it has nothing to do with food.

THE POWER
OF POSITIVE THINKING

Bonny and his family had only been in America a
few months when an old man approached them in
a shopping mall.

"You're nothing but a bunch of brown monkeys!"
the man said.

Bonny was unsure how to react. In the
Philippines, a public insult usually resulted in
somebody getting punched. But Bonny hated
violence. As a child he ran away from other boys

who bullied him, going off to cry alone -- which only made them taunt him more.

He didn't want to hit this man, but he didn't want to appear wounded, either, especially in front of his children. They were in a new country full of new possibilities. He didn't want them to be cautious and defensive as they started their new lives together.

So he decided to try out a new approach:

"I smiled and thanked him for the compliment," Bonny said.

"Since then, all the white people I have been meeting would smile at me. That old white man must have been telling all people like him to treat us brown monkeys nicely always. How lucky can some people ever get?"

Positivity is an important trait that Dr. Colberg identifies in her book, *50 Secrets of the Longest Living People with Diabetes*.

"Having a positive attitude is one of the key secrets to living well with diabetes, avoiding depression, and feeling happy overall," Colberg writes, citing a study from the University of North

Carolina at Chapel Hill showing that pessimists have a 42 percent higher death rate – from all causes, not just diabetes – than optimists.

For years, Bonny has often signed his emails as well as his posts on diabetes forums with the phrase "Enjoy life always!" It's a concept he learned from the late Rev. Norman Vincent Peale, whom Bonny heard speak twice in one day at two different churches Peale visited in the Philippines in the early 1960s

"What I heard from him definitely has been reminding me to always look at the bright side of life," Bonny says. "In one sermon, he talked about a flower growing out of barren ground in Korea where many Americans and Koreans had died. In the other sermon, he said that people keep on talking about places where they want to live. Most preferred peaceful places. But nobody ever wanted to live in the most peaceful places that are everywhere: the cemeteries."

Though Bonny and Nemia had their share of struggles in their new life in America, they refused to be defined by their problems, always believing that something good was right around the corner. And more often than not, they were right.

Though they were devastated to learn that Arnold had Duchenne Muscular Dystrophy, his courage as he battled his disease inspired his own family as well as everyone else he came in contact with.

When Nemia lost her job at Union Carbide in 1986, it wasn't long before she found a new position at the Dow Chemical Company in Midland, Mich.

Though Bonny would not necessarily have chosen to be diagnosed with type 2 diabetes, he knows that he is healthier and happier now than if he had continued on the path he was on, without adjusting his diet and exercise to compensate.

All along the way, he and Nemia were amazed how much people were willing to help them when they needed help. And when they had the opportunity, they helped others as much as they could.

"Every little thing that Nemia and I are able to do to make others happy definitely makes us enjoy life more," Bonny says.

From 1999 to 2001, Bonny and two classmates arranged for more than 100 unemployed, poverty-stricken Filipinos to come to the United States to take on seasonal jobs at Mackinac Island in Michigan and at a resort in Colorado Springs. Many of these workers were descendants of Bonny's aunts – the children and grandchildren of his father's three sisters who never received their share of the family inheritance his father had squandered.

"This was payback time for me," Bonny said.

This was the only definition of that term he was interested in. He knew from long experience in battle on the chessboard that revenge is a poor motive for any action, one that rarely pays off in the end.

Getting drawn into an argument with the old man who called him a "brown monkey" in 1973 would have done no good and likely would have caused more problems than the careless insult warranted. His children might have come away from the experience viewing others with suspicion instead of seeing the potential for good in meeting someone new.

In his 81 years, Bonny has learned that you cannot control others' behavior. But he can choose whether to focus on the good or the bad things in life.

"During winter, I hear many people say, 'I hate winter' or 'I hate these super-cold temperatures.' When I hear these complaints, I say to myself, 'Why complain about things I cannot control? What good do I get by complaining?'

"I think I am better off staying positive, cheerful, and busy doing something beneficial to me as well as to others."

The more that he works at this, the more he is able to live up to the saying under his name on diabetes forum postings: "Enjoy Life Always!"

V. AN UNCONVENTIONAL TYPE 2 PIONEER

WHY IT'S SMART TO ACT DUMB

If you ask Bonny the keys to his success in taming diabetes, he will tell you it's because he's DUMB, lazy and selfish.

Those obviously aren't characteristics that one usually associates with a pioneer. But then Bonny rarely sees things the way other people do.

DUMB is an acronym Bonny uses to remind himself to be "disciplined, upbeat, motivated, and bold."

"It just came to me out of the blue about 10 years ago," he says. "During this time I was actively defending my very controversial way of treating my diabetes at DLife.com." Though there were other people who were exercising, most were into low carb, high fat diets. "All of them were doing things very differently from what I did."

Not surprisingly, some of the people using the forum thought Bonny's ideas on treating his diabetes were dumb in the more conventional sense of the word. Instead of backing down, Bonny embraced the term. He wrote "DUMBT2D" under his name when he posted comments on the forum. At one point he even put it on his license plate.

Once again, Bonny found himself cast in the role of an outsider. He was used to people thinking he was weird, eccentric or just plain crazy. When he was young and poor growing up in the Philippines, it bothered him to feel like he didn't fit in. But now it is a role he cultivates and uses for his own benefit – and hopefully, others' as well.

Is there something unusual about his brain wiring, reflected in the fact that he is somewhat ambidextrous, a lefthander who learned to write with his right hand and now uses whichever hand is most convenient for many tasks, including using a computer mouse?

Is it because he grew up with an unusual name that people were always commenting on? He was proud of the name Damocles, which was unique in a country where most surnames were Spanish. He loved it when people asked him about "The Sword of Damocles." His first name, Bonaparte, was too grandiose for him, conjuring up the image of the conquering French hero Napoleon Bonaparte. Shortening it to Bonny sounded like a girl's name. He changed the spelling from the more feminine "Bonnie," but it was impossible to stop the teasing. So he simply embraced it, making people laugh by telling them he used to be a girl and then reminding them of the song "My Bonnie Lies Over the Ocean."

Now Bonny likes to keep a list in his head of all the things that make him unusual, such as the fact that he and his wife don't wear wedding rings because at the time they married they were far too poor to afford them. At the top of the list is his unusual method of treating his diabetes, from his stair running to his generous consumption of carbohydrates.

Some people think stair climbing is a dumb way to exercise. Bonny couldn't agree more. He is **disciplined** about getting in four short periods of exercise each day, **upbeat** in his approach,

motivated to stick with it and **bold** enough to share his ideas with others. It all adds up to a textbook example of acting DUMB.

Never content to stick with the status quo, however, Bonny recently decided to change his acronym.

"I promoted myself from DUMB to DUMBEST," he said.

So now his new goals are to be:

Disciplined
Upbeat
Motivated
Bold
Empowered
Sensible
Tough.

It's the best way he knows to keep his diabetes under control.

EXERCISE LIKE CRAZY
SO YOU CAN BE LAZY

Media coverage of Bonny over the years inevitably makes him sound like an outlier who pushes himself far beyond what ordinary people with type 2 diabetes could ever accomplish.

Diabetes Forecast magazine cited Bonny's "extreme approach to fitness" in a July 2010 profile chronicling what was then a two-hour daily regimen of stair running. It might sound crazy to some people, the writer noted, "but an intense exercise routine is how he's been able to manage type 2 diabetes for most of 19 years without medication."

A 2015 article in *Diabetes Health* magazine compared his pre-meal workouts to those of a lion: He "exercises at the first sign of hunger," replicating the wild beast's need to hunt for its food rather than simply opening the refrigerator.

Even Dr. Sheri R. Colberg, who advocates rigorous exercise as part of diabetes care, expressed surprise at the intensity of Bonny's workouts when she responded to an email in 2016, congratulating him on reaching the milestone of 25 years without using medication.

"That's great that you've been able to keep up that regimen for 25 years," she wrote, noting that she had never heard of anyone with type 2 diabetes going so long without using drugs or suffering complications. "Most people would get injured or demotivated with such a stringent training regimen and time commitment."

But what Colberg and others don't realize is that Bonny doesn't run stairs because he's a shard-core athlete or a glutton for punishment.

He does it because he's lazy.

"I have always been lazy all my life," he says. "I don't work as hard as others do. Why? Because I am very good at finding shortcuts."

The way Bonny sees it, climbing the stairs is the ultimate shortcut because it's the quickest and cheapest way to raise his heart rate enough to clear his blood of excess sugar.

Not driving somewhere else to exercise saves him time he could spend doing something else he'd rather be doing, like playing chess.

Not spending money on a gym membership, exercise equipment, workout clothes or even shoes – he typically climbs the stairs barefoot or in socks – frees up his budget for other things.

Once he made stair climbing part of his routine, it became automatic. He didn't have to think about it, other than periodically reviewing whether there was a way to do it even more quickly and easily.

Over time, he learned to run the stairs only as long as was necessary to bring his blood sugar down into the normal range after meals. He went from two hours of stair running per day to 100 minutes, broken up into four blocks of 25 minutes each. In more recent years he has switched to four blocks of 15 minutes for 60 total minutes.

In 2016, he wondered what would happen if he tried walking the stairs instead of running. When his October A1C test registered 5.8 percent – the same as his test six months earlier – he decided there was no point in running when he could walk much more safely and easily. (He takes the steps two at a time to increase the difficulty level, and descends the stairs backward, which is easier on his knees.)

Bonny continues to refine his exercise routine to make it as simple and efficient as possible. Because he exults in his own special brand of laziness, spending as much time as possible doing exactly as he wants, he is always looking for ways to get better results with less work.

The more he looks for shortcuts, the more he finds. If he were just starting out now, Bonny says he would probably try a High Intensity Interval Training workout. Studies have shown that these HIIT workouts, as they are known, deliver good results in a short amount of time.

One popular HIIT program that was originally published in the American College of Sports Medicine's Health & Fitness Journal in 2013 has been said to essentially pack the benefits of going for a run and visiting a weight room into seven minutes of exercise. It is easy to find online if you Google "Scientific 7-MinuteWorkout."

More recently, scientists at McMaster University in Hamilton, Ontario, came out with a study showing that one minute of strenuous exercise provides as much benefit as 45 minutes of moderate exercise. That study has since led to a book that came out in early 2017 called *The One-Minute Workout*.

Bonny tweaks his exercise program from time to time based on ideas he comes across in his reading – though as a proponent of the Three E's (see Page 82), he might well question why an entire book was needed to explain a one-minute exercise program.

Nonetheless, he sees no need to abandon a highly successful exercise routine that has generated proven results over nearly 26 years.

Now, at an age when many people – whether or not they have diabetes – fear their bodies are breaking down, Bonny feels confident in his health even as he looks for ways to improve it.

So far, being lazy seems to be working out for him.

WHY IT'S GOOD TO BE SELFISH

Bonny once received an award for being selfish.

That's the way he looks at it. Officially, he was awarded the Mapa Blue Falcon Award for Humanitarian Service from his old high school in the Philippines a few years ago for helping others. But the secret behind his acts of kindness is pure selfishness: He does it because it makes him feel good.

The more Bonny helps people, the better he feels. In the end, even though he is helping others at his expense, he gets the biggest payoff of all because the whole process feeds his ego and improves his self-esteem.

Bonny believes that playing chess helps him hone this perspective, because the more he learns to appreciate the game, the less fixated he is on whether he wins or loses. Playing chess has taught him not to be angry when he loses – not at his opponent and not at himself, either. There is always something to be learned from a loss on the chessboard. Getting angry gets in the way of learning those important lessons. The more he plays, the more he learns – not just about chess, but about life.

Much as the internet changed Bonny's life by making it possible to learn what other people with diabetes were thinking and doing to manage their disease, it was even more exciting when he discovered an online site of chess enthusiasts from around the world. At any moment of any day, there was always someone, somewhere, who was ready to play.

And as a retiree who worked hard at setting up his daily routine to spend as little time as possible on the necessary tasks of daily living, Bonny was almost always ready. He can, and does, spend hours every day playing chess.

Is he being selfish?

"The time I used up playing hundreds of online chess games every day is time I could have used on something more important," Bonny admits.

He knows that's what his wife thinks, because she frequently says so.

A similar debate often comes up on fitness forums, whose members must grapple with guilt over whether they're taking too much time away from their spouses and families by devoting so much time to exercise. Training for a marathon or a 100-mile bike race can take almost as much time as a part-time job, and that doesn't include the travel time and expense of getting to the event itself, which may be in another city or even another state.

These fitness buffs may be enjoying the best health of their adult lives, with energy levels they haven't experienced in decades. In the long term, the work they're doing gives them *more* time with their families because they're reducing the possibility of an untimely death. Their renewed energy may translate into getting more work done around the house and more time spent playing with their children.

But in the short term, after the initial excitement over a big weight loss or other health improvement wears off, family members may feel that their loved ones are being selfish by spending so much time staying fit.

Worrying about whether his exercise program is taking time away from his family has never been an issue for Bonny. To avoid the expense, hassle and possible side effects of medication, Bonny must raise his heart rate to keep his blood sugar in check. From the very beginning of his life as a type 2 diabetic, he knew he had to exercise at home in case his son Arnold needed him. Then, when Nemia had a stroke shortly after Arnold's death in 1999, Bonny had to exercise at home in case Nemia needed his help.

Though Nemia recovered well enough to return to work a few months later, she still has more difficulty walking than she used to. In all the years since, Bonny has continued to exercise at home, in part to stay near Nemia but also because he simply prefers exercising at home. In retirement, Nemia had adopted a similar version of Bonny's exercise program, doing many of the same exercises but walking around the house rather than up the stairs as a safety precaution.

Chess, however, is another matter. Bonny firmly believes that playing chess makes him a better person, and by extension, a better husband.

"If chess really does make me a better, more understanding, more loving and more helpful person," he reasons, "then others will definitely benefit from my being so."

However, like the spouses of many fitness enthusiasts, it is hard for Nemia to watch Bonny devote hours and hours to online chess without feeling like he could surely be doing something more productive.

Bonny's solution to their difference of opinion on this matter, as always, is to defer to his wife's wishes.

"Every time Nem wants something, she gets it," he says. "There's no point in contradicting her. Both of us very well know that our marriage is forever and there will never be a divorce or separation. I strongly believe that there is no better wife for me. I surely got the best one for me."

That being the case, he says, "I am duty-bound to make myself the best husband for her. I can control only myself, and I very well know that I cannot control others."

So even though Bonny could easily justify in his own mind online chess marathons that last for hours, he plays chess only during times when Nemia is busy doing other things. They may disagree as to whether online chess is always the most meaningful use of his time, but as long as she doesn't have to dwell on the image of him at his virtual chessboard, it is less of an issue.

Sometimes, despite 59 years of devoting himself to making his wife happy, Bonny still makes mistakes and manages to upset her. When this happens, he makes sure he is the one who gives in.

"I learned very easily that it is easier for me to forgive and forget than to wait for her to forgive me and forget a bad exchange of words. She does not forget, unfortunately."

But Bonny doesn't dwell on mistakes. In his mind, fretting over something he did wrong is the biggest time waster of all. Instead, he says, "I spend more time and effort on being kind, generous, understanding, forgiving, caring, loving, listening more and talking less."

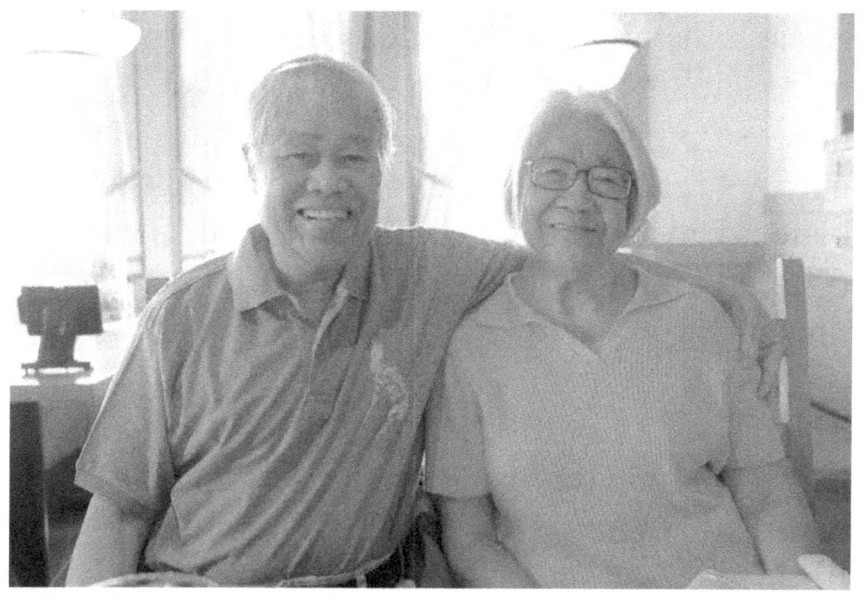

Bonny and Nemia in 2017, a few weeks before their 59th wedding anniversary.

Why? Because he is selfish.

This isn't necessarily something that the youthful Bonny would have read in the newspaper in the quotes of wisdom section. He admits it's part of his own peculiar viewpoint. Nonetheless, he feels very strongly that human beings were designed to be selfish – for a good cause.

His explanation: "Everything I do, like being nice, generous and kind to others is always for my own good. If I help somebody, I feel good."

Because he remains convinced that his wife is more intelligent than he is, "that forces me to never stop improving myself in every way I can. I may not reach her level, but doing my best to be better keeps me occupied full time. This means that petty things are not worth my attention and time."

The ultimate payoff? "Being loyal, loving and caring to my wife for 59 years gives me the feeling that I know the secret of enjoying a good life."

He sees sharing what he's learned about diabetes with others as a similar selfish act with a good payoff.

"If I succeed in helping future type 2 diabetics to have a good, healthy, productive and happy life like mine," he says, "that surely is good for my ego."

VI. EMBRACING THE FUTURE

DIABETES, THE GREAT EQUALIZER

Bonny limits himself to one hour of TV per day, which he typically watches while standing in the kitchen, eating his evening meal.

Since his diagnosis, he rarely sits unless he's at the computer or dining with guests or in a restaurant. When members of his chess club gather at his home for their weekly meeting, he plays game after game standing up. When he has company, he invites his guests to take the most comfortable seats in the room, but he never bothers to sit himself, conducting even the lengthiest conversations on his feet.

By the time Bonny turned on the TV on Feb. 5, 2017, Super Bowl LI was already well into the third quarter. He missed most of the multicultural commercials that generated a great deal of buzz on social media.

As a Filipino immigrant, Bonny might have been pleased by the ads that showed Americans of all skin tones and ethnicities in a positive, unifying light – though as a type 2 diabetic who has drunk nothing but water since July 1991, he could never support the underlying theme in the Coca-Cola ad that all Americans should celebrate by drinking sugary soda.

It's too bad the American Diabetes Association didn't run a Super Bowl commercial pointing out the risk factors for the people portrayed on the screen – a timely reminder on a day renowned for gluttony.

Unfortunately, type 2 diabetes is one case in which all Americans are *not* created equal. Certain ethnic groups have a much higher risk than others. There is one unifying factor, however, that affects Americans of every skin tone: the rates are rising all across the land, from sea to shining sea.

Bonny is well aware of the risk facing Filipino-Americans.

"When I was newly diagnosed, I found out very easily that out of 2,000-plus of us who graduated from our high school in 1955, most of us who went overseas to Canada and the U.S.A. became type 2s," he said.

Among those who stayed in the Philippines, it seemed like only those who were wealthy became diabetic. This included Bonny's cousin, who became vice president of the refrigerator company Bonny worked with on his export business. His cousin's wife and oldest son became diabetic as well.

"I have this strong suspicion that only smart people get type 2 diabetes" in the Philippines, he says. "How is that? Type 2 diabetes is caused by inactivity plus too much food consumption. Poor people have no choice but to stay active all the time looking for food which they don't have."

Bonny can't help suspecting that immigrants from other poor countries face a similar fate.

"The moment they did well in life by working very hard, they easily learn to overeat and watch TV lying down and munching something most of the time."

That was the case with him. Unlearning this behavior – going back to a diet that is now much more like what he was used to eating as a poor Asian – has helped him keep his disease in check. Because he cannot easily replicate the exercise he got in Manila, walking everywhere with no car, he has had to manufacture a replacement exercise program.

"In my early years as a diabetic, the story going around was about the American Indians. These were people who hunted for their survival." Now, with a much more sedentary lifestyle, Native Americans have among the highest type 2 diabetes rates in the nation.

The reality, however, is that all Americans, regardless of race, are increasingly in danger of developing diabetes as obesity rates rise and sedentary lifestyles prevail. Though the risk varies among different ethnic groups, diabetes has essentially become the Great Equalizer in American society, a country so wealthy that even most of those who live in poverty nonetheless manage to consume too many calories and get too little exercise.

According to the American Diabetes Association, the economic cost of type 2 diabetes in this country alone is now more than $245 billion a year. Around the globe, urbanization and industrialization are creating "high-carbon obesogenic environments" dependent on cars and convenience foods, accelerating the risk – and costs – of diabetes worldwide, according to the International Diabetes Federation.

These days Bonny encounters many people of all skin colors with type 2 diabetes – friends, relatives, neighbors, members of his chess club. Some are doctors who seem just as helpless as their patients when it comes to helping themselves or family members with the disease.

Bonny wishes others would realize how simple it really is to control type 2 diabetes. But he doesn't like to make recommendations to others, and he doubts whether most people would listen even if he tried.

"I don't give advice," he says. "People are very sensitive. I feel that nobody accepts that somebody else is better than him.

"I am different. I know people who are superior to me, and others who are inferior to me. I learn something from all of them."

NEVER STOP ENJOYING LIFE

Back in 1955, Bonny could hardly believe he had
the good fortune to participate in the First
National Junior Chess Championship in Manila.

If he had known then that 59 years later, he would
not only compete against the runner-up of that
tournament at his home in America, but that he
would win one of their matches, he would have
found that very hard to believe.

"I got lucky," he says of his win against Jose
Hilado, who became an accountant who wound up

in Toronto. "I got him in time control. Without the clock, he was the sure winner."

Bonny does not consider himself to be particularly good at chess. "My rating now of 1600 means that I am just an average chess player," he says.

Nonetheless, he is often able to defeat superior players in timed games by using the clock to his advantage. During one recent meeting of the Midland Chess Club, for example, he beat a young executive from the Dow Chemical Company four out of five games.

"I won because he kept on running out of time. If there was no time limit, I would have lost all five games."

The secret to Blitz games, Bonny explains, "is to confuse your opponent so that he will be forced to waste his time figuring out how to solve an unfamiliar position."

The ability to adapt to changing circumstances is important in chess. It is this same ability to adapt that has made it possible for Bonny to stay healthy and active into his 80s, nearly 26 years after being diagnosed with type 2 diabetes.

At the time of his diagnosis, it might have been easy to feel overwhelmed. At 55, he was caring for an adult son with a fatal disease. His mother was suffering from Alzheimer's. And now he had a disease of his own to worry about.

There would be many difficulties ahead. Both his youngest son and his mother would die within a year of each other in the late 1990s. Then, just a month after Arnold's death, Nemia would suffer a stroke. She would eventually return to work, but she would never fully recover, having to walk much more slowly from that point on.

Still, there were many good things that lay in his future as well. In 1995 he returned to the Philippines for his 40th high school reunion.

"Meeting my high school classmates after 40 years of separation from each other, most of our conversations made me feel that we never got separated. It really was just like we were still in high school," he said.

That's how he felt, anyway. Some of his friends were not in good health. One boy who used to walk home from school with him was now a man with a heart problem that made him too ill to attend the reunion. Bonny and another friend left the party to surprise him, arriving at his home while he was in the shower. Prompted by his classmate's wife, Bonny said something to his friend through the bathroom door and was surprised that his old friend recognized his voice.

"Bonny, you are the guy I want to see," his friend replied, emerging from the bathroom.

Later that night, Bonny was among eight classmates now living in the U.S. and Canada who were asked to speak a few words. Once again, despite the problems he was dealing with back home, he was reminded of his good fortune. The high school student who had once been so poor he often had no lunch realized that the money he earned in America could buy much more in the Philippines.

Over the years Bonny found ways to help those from his old school, sending money to help cover the costs of Christmas parties so more of his classmates could afford to attend. To celebrate the 50th anniversary of his high school graduation, he and Nemia provided scholarship money for eight 2005 graduates of Mapa High School to attend Polytechnic University of the Philippines, formerly known as the Philippine College of

Commerce, where Bonny began his own college studies.

"Two of our scholars finished five-year electrical engineering courses, five finished four-year degree courses, and one quit after her sophomore year," Bonny said.

For his efforts, Bonny's former high school later awarded him the Mapa Blue Falcon Award for Humanitarian Service. He took special pleasure in learning he was the 33rd recipient of this award. Bonny's father had once told him that 33 was not only the age of Jesus Christ when he was nailed to the cross, but the highest rank that a Free Mason can earn. Bonny's father was never able to earn enough money to help himself or his family, but he admired this secret order for their good works.

"He told me that they do good things for their members and for others who need help, and they never talk about them," Bonny said.

Bonny never became a Free Mason. But he enjoyed quietly doing things to help others. And he loved watching for the number 33. He graduated 33rd out of 2,000 in his high school class. When he came to the United States, he found it in his Social Security number and on his license plate. And now, it seemed especially symbolic in connection to an award for his quiet way of helping others.

In 2011, Bonny had the pleasure of hosting his old friend Diwang at his home in Midland. Though they had kept in touch, and always saw each other on Bonny's return trips to the Philippines, it was Diwang's first trip to America since a 1960 sightseeing tour on his way back from a year of study in the United Kingdom.

"I lost the only chess game we played during his visit," Bonny says. But he took solace in his friend's joy at winning both that match and another on his trip, against a former subordinate from the Manila City Engineer's Office who now lives in Toronto. "Both games he won made him truly happy."

Bonny was glad for his friend. Though he didn't know it at the time, he would never see Diwang again. He died two years later, in 2013.

Though Bonny missed his 50th class reunion in 2005 due to a bad case of the flu, there would be other get-togethers with former classmates in the U.S. and Canada. It was on one of these mini reunions, in Niagara Falls, that he met a fellow chess enthusiast from Toronto who has since become a good friend, Oliver Kilayko.

In 2014, Kilayko and his wife came to visit Bonny and Nemia in Midland. Accompanying them were another Toronto couple: Kilayko's cousin, Jose Hilado, who happened to be the 1955 runner-up at the First National Junior Chess Championship in Manila.

They played a lot of chess that weekend, and the group stayed through Monday night so they could participate in the weekly meeting of the Midland Chess Club. Bonny was thrilled when he managed to defeat Hilado.

It took him 59 years to do it, but not only had he managed to beat the 1955 runner-up but also the 1956 tournament champion, as Hilado went on to win the following year.

"We had a very good time," Bonny said. And it might never have happened if he hadn't made a commitment to manage his diabetes in the simplest way possible, relying on diet and exercise rather than drugs.

Even now, at 81, Bonny sees no reason to quit the regimen that has kept him happy and healthy all

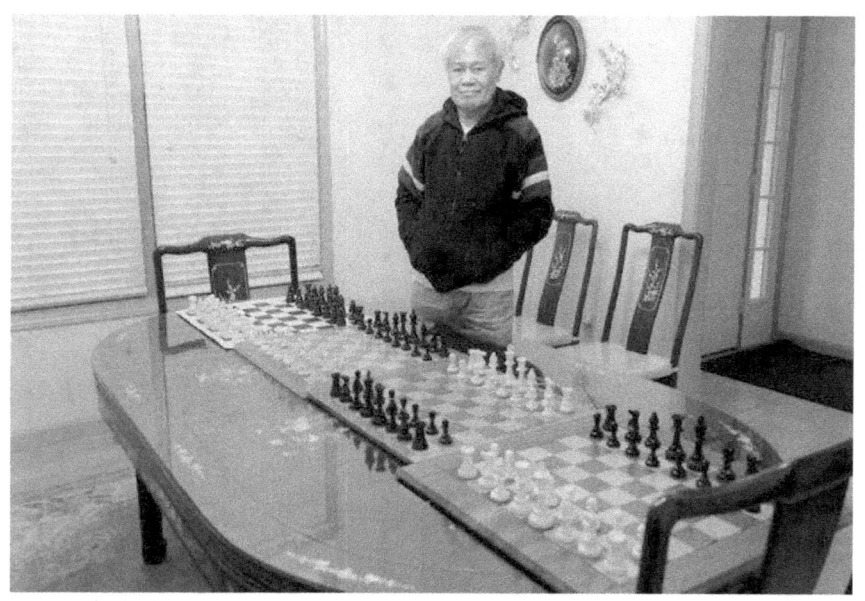

When his chess-loving friends come to visit, Bonny will sometimes set up multiple chessboards so they can play four games at once.

these years. Though he doesn't have a "bucket list" with goals he wants to cross off in the years ahead, he is determined to make it to age 100 – or, as he might view it, three times 33, plus one.

Along the way he intends to never stop enjoying life, to take pleasure in the things that please him and to appreciate whatever comes his way.

And with this book, he hopes to help others do the same.

APPENDIX

The Arnold Dance

This is the exercise routine that Bonny did while his son Arnold was hospitalized with Duchenne Muscular Dystrophy in the 1990s. Unable to complete his usual exercise routine of jogging up the stairs in his home, Bonny came up with the following way to raise his heart rate enough to keep his blood sugar levels under control.

To warm up, as well as for a cool down afterward, Bonny would lift his legs one at a time, shaking them in all directions for a few moments.

Then he would begin the following routine, starting slowly and then going faster and faster, but never getting out of control to the point that he might fall or hurt himself. The arm motions and leg motions are done simultaneously:

1. First, bend both arms at the elbow to make 90-degree angles.

2. Second, clench your fists and begin moving your arms forward and backward.

3. Now, while continuing to move your arms, bend your knees and go down into a squat position, as low as you can comfortably go, before returning to a standing position.

   Breathe deeply, exhaling as you move.

4. After two to three minutes of this activity, stop and switch to jogging in place for as long as you can comfortably do so, up to three or four minutes if possible.

5. Now, alternate back and forth between the squatting motion activity and jogging in place, checking to see whether your heart rate is in the appropriate range recommended for exercise. (An easy way to do this is to take your pulse at your wrist for 10 seconds, then multiply the number of heartbeats counted by six.)

If you feel dizzy or lightheaded, stop immediately. Otherwise, continue alternating between the squatting motion and jogging in place for a minimum of 10 minutes, or more if desired.

Bonny in the Kitchen

Shortly before Bonny and his children left the Philippines for America in October 1972, he met with the American husband of a good friend. Among his many questions about life in the United States was an inquiry about the availability and cost of maids.

In the Philippines, with both Bonny and Nemia working full-time, they had relied on up to three maids at one time to help with the cooking, cleaning and children. In Manila, household help was top quality and yet very inexpensive.

"Countries all over the world employ Filipino maids," Bonny says. "They are efficient, clean, good, and cheap. There are many American retirees in the Philippines and one of the reasons they are there is the availability of cheap maids."

Things were different in America, his friend's husband told him. Maids in the United States tended to be from Spanish-speaking countries, and they cost much more than what Bonny and Nemia were used to paying. On the other hand, the affordability of electric and gas appliances made housework in American homes much less time consuming. There was no need to wash clothes by hand, the man said, explaining how his family simply threw laundry in a washing machine. Microwaves and gas ovens made cooking food much easier as well.

When Bonny began working from home and caring for Arnold after their move to Michigan in 1986, he applied his "Three E's" methodology to household tasks such as cleaning and laundry. However, he never really learned to cook. If there was no leftover food from another meal, he went out to buy carryout meals for Nemia and Arnold while preparing something simple for himself, such as boiled eggs or baked fish.

Though Nemia has done most of the cooking since she retired in 2004, Bonny will on occasion prepare food for himself if needed.

"If I do the cooking, it should be the easiest and fastest way," he says. With vegetables, for instance, this typically means eating them either boiled or fresh.

"If I want to eat it fresh, I wash it more than once and then immerse it in vinegar and then rinse it."

Bonny and Nemia's refrigerator is not cluttered with endless jars of sauces and toppings. The flavoring they use most often is fish sauce, a staple in many Filipino homes that is added to meat-and-vegetable dishes.

Also missing from their refrigerator: the ubiquitous gallon of milk. Bonny drinks only water. If milk is needed in a recipe, such as the banana bread he sometimes bakes, they use evaporated milk which can be stored in a cupboard until it is needed.

Both refrigerator and cupboard contain only the foods that Bonny and Nemia consume on a regular basis. A crisper drawer in the refrigerator one afternoon in autumn 2016, for instance, was filled with avocados purchased on sale. Shelves in the cupboard were lined with jars of natural peanut butter and sugar-free fruit cocktail, for times when they may run low on fresh fruits.

Bonny does very little baking. In recent years there are only two types of baked goods he has prepared on an occasional basis, both as a means of getting the 100 percent dark cocoa powder he includes in his diet to help control his blood pressure. He will also stir cocoa powder into oatmeal.

These recipes are listed below, though he cautions readers that he eats "for nutrition, not taste."

Bonny's dark chocolate banana bread

(Adapted from a recipe he found on Dr. Ben Kim's website, drbenkim.com)

4 eggs
1 cup evaporated milk
2 tbsp extra virgin olive oil
4 mashed ripe bananas
1 cup chopped walnuts
2 1/2 cups whole wheat flour
1 tbsp baking power
1 tsp. cinnamon
1 cup raisins
1 cup 100 percent dark chocolate cocoa powder
1 cup water

Directions:

1) Preheat oven to 350 degrees. Lightly grease two 4" x 8" bread pans
2) Combine eggs, evaporated milk, oil, water, and mashed bananas in a bowl and mix until homogenized. Set aside.
3) Mix flour, baking powder, cinnamon and cocoa powder.
4) Add wet ingredients and gently stir to form batter.
5) Gently fold in raisins and walnuts.
6) Pour batter into baking pans.
7) Bake for about 55 minutes.

Banana oat cookies

2 mashed bananas mixed with 1 teaspoon each of vanilla and cinnamon
1 cup raisins
2 cups oats
1 cup chopped walnuts
½ cup cocoa powder
2 cups water

Pour batter in an 8 1/2" x 8 1/2" pan. Bake 20 minutes at 350 degrees.

Nemia's Biko
(sweet rice pudding)

Nemia learned to cook from her mother when she was growing up in Isabela, a province located in the northern part of Luzon, the largest island in the Philippines. (Manila is located in the central part of Luzon.)

Biko is a popular Filipino dessert made with glutinous rice, also known as sticky rice or "malagkit na bigas" in Tagalog, the primary Filipino language spoken along with English in the Philippines.

Ingredients:
1 14-oz can sweetened condensed milk
1 14 oz can coconut milk
4 cups sweet rice
Water, as needed (see below)
1) Use a rice cooker. Mix 4 cups of rice, water and coconut milk, making sure that the total amount of water and milk is 6 cups.

2) Once the rice is cooked, put it in a mixing container. Mix the condensed milk and the rice. It may be necessary to add some water to facilitate mixing.

3) Put the mixed rice and condensed milk in a pan and bake it for 20-25 minutes at 350 degrees.

Exercise Case Study: Bonny Damocles

The following article was published July 2010 in Diabetes Forecast magazine and online at http://www.diabetesforecast.org/2010/jul/exercise -case-study-bonny-damocles.html.

Diabetes Forecast 2010

The following is reprinted with permission from the American Diabetes Association:

By Erika Gebel, PhD
July 2010

Running up and down a flight of stairs for a total of two hours every day, Bonny Damocles, 74, has taken an extreme approach to fitness. But an intense exercise routine is how he's been able to manage type 2 diabetes for most of 19 years without medication.

Damocles, an engineer from Midland, Mich., emigrated from the Philippines to the United States with his wife, Nemia, in 1978. "Moving from a poor country to a wealthy country, we had a chance to enjoy all the 'good things' this country offers," says Damocles, meaning lots of fast food and no exercise. "We practically didn't move."

He went from a svelte 126 pounds on his 5-foot, 7-inch frame to a heftier 165. Then, in July 1991, Damocles lost a pound a day for two straight weeks. "I thought I had cancer," he recalls.

A trip to his family physician revealed that his blood glucose level was 468 mg/dl. The diagnosis was type 2 diabetes. The doctor wanted to start him on oral medications immediately, but Damocles balked. "I begged him to give me a few days to try something else," he says.

Damocles and his doctor made a deal. He had two weeks to rein in his blood glucose. If it didn't drastically improve, he would start the medication. Damocles was on a mission.

"In 10 days of running our stairs a daily total of two hours, my sugar readings were already in the 130s," says Damocles. At the same time, Damocles dramatically changed his eating habits, going from a fast-food-friendly diet to one grounded in fruits, vegetables, grains, seeds, nuts, beans, and seaweed. "The first 10 days of my diabetic life clearly proved to me that I could confidently depend on my exercise routine as my only diabetes medication."

Could most people avoid or stop taking diabetes meds by clocking two hours of stair-running a day? Research has shown that lifestyle changes can often halt pre-diabetes in its tracks, but it's less clear whether people with type 2 can typically control blood glucose over the long term through diet and exercise alone. Plus, for many people, repetitive strain injuries might make a Damocles-like routine unsustainable. "People who tried to duplicate what I did, well, most of them got in big trouble," says Damocles. "They ended up having knee problems."

Even for him, the routine was difficult, and after a while, Damocles began to wonder if such extremes were still necessary. "After four years, my exercise routine was so effective, I felt cured. All my readings were normal," he says. "For the next 3 1/2 years, I sort of went back to my old self."

But Damocles was not cured, and after a few years of little exercise, his blood glucose levels crept back up. He didn't know how bad it had gotten until he was tested and saw that his blood glucose was again in the 400s. "That was a warning," he says. "Since then, I really became dedicated to taking good care of myself and went back to two hours a day."

Damocles says he is now free of diabetes complications. His knees started bothering him recently; he's not sure if the culprit is overuse, old age, or both. So, he's replaced stair-running with lower-impact exercises like running in place and strength training. So far, he's been able to control his diabetes with this new approach; the A1C (average blood glucose over the past two to three months) from his last checkup was 5.8 percent, well within the range of 7 percent or less recommended for people with diabetes by the American Diabetes Association.

Damocles doesn't recommend his unusual style of diabetes management to everyone, and indeed, it's important to check with a doctor before making big changes in your fitness routine. "My motivation is that me and my wife would like to reach 100 years old," says Damocles. "If you have that kind of goal, you have to be disciplined."

AN 80-YEAR-OLD'S WORKOUT KICKS MY BUTT

The following is a blog post written by co-author Tanya Isch Caylor and published at https://90in9.wordpress.com *on May 16, 2016:*

When a guy I interviewed recently for a diabetes magazine told me he controls his blood sugar with daily stair-running, I couldn't resist giving his workout a try.

Having recently climbed the steps up a 25-story skyscraper without pausing to catch my breath, I figured I was up for the challenge – especially considering the guy I was writing about is 80 years old.

Bonny Damocles told me he runs up and down a single flight of 16 steps in his house for a total of 100 minutes, broken up into 4 sets of 25 minutes.

Using our 12-step stairway, I stopped running after 3 minutes and began to walk. I finished that first 25-minute set, and managed to do three more sets over the course of the day, but except for a couple of minutes at the beginning of each, I had to settle for walking up the steps.

The difficulty here is that in addition to the lung-busting component, running stairs is mind-numbingly dull unless you are listening to a really riveting book on tape (which is what helped me get through sets 2-4. Thank you, Jonathan Kellerman).

So what's the secret to Bonny's mental toughness? For starters, a profound desire to avoid taking medication to control his type 2 diabetes. He's coming up on 25 years since his diagnosis and says he's in excellent health with no complications from the disease. That takes an extraordinary amount of willpower and dedication to a hardcore fitness program. As a guy who sometimes went days at a time without food growing up in the Philippines during World War II, Bonny definitely has a survivor's mindset. Running stairs was the toughest – and cheapest –

form of exercise he could think of. When it brought his blood sugar down from over 400 to 130 in 10 days, convincing his doctor he could continue his regimen without meds, Bonny's course was set. (It doesn't hurt that he's not a very big guy, carrying 139 pounds on a 5-7 frame, so he has less mass to haul up those stairs.)

I really HATE this workout. And yet I now find myself doing it at least once a week. As somebody who primarily works from home, it's appealing to have tough workouts that I can do even when I think I don't have time. Fitting in 15 minutes here and there gets me past those points in the day when I feel momentarily "stuck." And I'm slowly starting to build up how many of those stairs I run up vs. walking.

So: Thanks, Bonny, for the inspiration. (I think.) :)

ABOUT THE AUTHORS

Tanya Isch Caylor is a health and fitness writer who lives in northeast Indiana with her husband, Bob, and two of their four children who are still at home. She is the author of *A Swiss Banker in Indiana Farm Country: How a Farm Boy Grew Up to Lead One of America's Most Efficient Banks.*

Bonny C. Damocles is a graduate of the Manuel L. Quezon University School of Engineering and Architecture and Mapa High School, which awarded him the Mapa Blue Falcon Award for Humanitarian Service in 2013. Both are located in Manila, the Philippines, where he spent the first 37 years of his life and worked as a management analyst in the Manila Mayor's Office. A retired businessman, he lives with his wife, Nemia, in Midland, Mich., where he is the weekly host of the Midland Chess Club.

www.ingramcontent.com/pod-product-compliance
Lightning Source LLC
Chambersburg PA
CBHW071341280526
45787CB00001B/166